Pediatric Home Companion

Commonsense Advice About Your Child's Health

LISA WISEMAN, M.D.

Quality Medical Publishing, Inc.

ST. LOUIS, MISSOURI
1997

Cover photo by Joe Hanig

This book is written to help you make informed decisions about your child's health
and to communicate with your physician more effectively. It is not intended to be used
as an in-depth review of illnesses, diagnoses, and treatments. Although care has been
taken to ensure that the information presented is as accurate and up to date as possible,
medical knowledge is constantly changing, and you should consult your physician
about current standards of practice.

Printed in the United States of America.

Quality Medical Publishing, Inc.
11970 Borman Drive, Suite 222
St. Louis, Missouri 63146

LIBRARY OF CONGRESS CATALOGING-IN-PUBLICATION DATA

Wiseman, Lisa.
        Pediatric home companion : commonsense advice about your child's
    health / Lisa Wiseman.
            p.   cm.
        Includes index.
        ISBN 1-57626-036-4
        1. Pediatrics—Popular works.   I. Title.
    RJ61.W815   1997
    618.92—dc21   97-22119
                                                                             CIP

QMP/IPC/IPC
5   4   3   2   1

To

my own pediatric home companions
Savannah, Marsy, and **James**

in loving memory of their
Aunt Polly
(1964-1996)

Preface

Pediatric Home Companion: Commonsense Advice About Your Child's Health is not just another encyclopedia of childhood illnesses and treatments. There are already enough of those lining the bookstore shelves. Rather it is written to address the most frequently asked questions by parents of healthy, normal children who seek simplified explanations for common pediatric problems. These same questions come up so often that it has become clear to me that the traditional "baby books" have failed to meet the needs of busy parents who are torn between the demands of the workplace and serving the best interests of an ailing child.

There is no substitute for a trusted pediatrician when your child is sick. These days, however, it is rare that the same pediatrician oversees the care of a child throughout childhood as jobs and insurance plans change. Unfortunately, medical care today has become so fragmented and specialized that much of the burden of medical decision making must be assumed by parents. Even well-informed parents have misconceptions that become obstacles to good health care for their child. Compounding the problem, health professionals have different opinions. Parents are so bombarded by information and misinformation from the media and well-intentioned in-laws, neighbors, and friends that sorting through it all can be difficult and frustrating.

Most parents want to be actively involved in their child's medical care, but they want to feel confident that they have asked all the right questions and have been given unhurried and complete answers. This book attempts to explain the pediatrician's rationale for making certain decisions and thus avoid expensive and time-consuming office visits that leave parents feeling frustrated and uncertain. Informed parents can participate in a more productive dialogue with pediatricians and can make intelligent decisions when they understand all the options.

Pediatric Home Companion is not organized in the traditional way by symptoms, diseases, or age groups. Chapter 1, "Your Healthy Child," sets the stage by discussing well-child issues such as nutrition and growth, the influence of education, sports, and music lessons on development, and routine well-child examinations. It is an unconventional approach that is more in keeping with the lifestyles of children in the nineties. The lastest information on the role of genetics and heredity is presented. (Your baby does come with an instruction manual; it's in his genes. If you are patient, he will read it to you himself.)

Chapter 2, "Getting Down to Basics," discusses concerns that parents of sick children have regardless of their age or illness. It addresses the question that plaques parents: How sick is sick? It also explains the role of fever and puts to rest the age-old myth that high fever causes brain damage and convulsions. Finally, the principles of contagiousness are presented so that a parent can decide when a child can safely return to day care or school and the caretaker to work.

Chapter 3 takes you on a tour of your medicine cabinet. This chapter covers common medications for typical childhood conditions and helps you understand what they can or cannot be expected to do so that you can intelligently medicate your child if indicated.

First-time mothers are the focus of Chapter 4 entitled "You and Your Newborn." It encourages new moms to relax and trust their instincts. Practical and realistic options for the feeding and care of your newborn are discussed in addition to common conditions that may alarm parents but are generally not serious. Those of us who have been there know that in retrospect it doesn't have to be as hard as we made it. Spend more time with your baby and less time reading the "how-to" books.

Chapter 5 is for those of you who feel like screaming when you hear, "It's *just* his allergies." Allergies won't kill you, but they might make you wish you were dead. The immune system that serves to protect the body is just doing its job too well. Allergic rhinitis and conjunctivitis, asthma, atopic dermatitis, and insect bites and stings are covered. There is a detailed discussion of the implications of the "penicillin allergic" label that is often needlessly applied.

Individual diseases and problems are the subject of Chapter 6. Although Chapters 1 to 5 dealt with many of the underlying principles involved in these prevalent conditions and their treatment, this is a handy reference that you may wish to consult on a frequent basis. This guide could help you determine whether a trip to the pediatrician is warranted or can help you anticipate what to expect when you do go.

The current issues relating to the increasingly complex immunization schedules are discussed in Chapter 7. Most parents are very receptive to immunizing their children, but the few who aren't can be downright militant in their opposition. I hope I can convince a few skeptics that required immunizations are not part of a federal subsidy program for pediatricians or an alien plot to destroy humanity. Immunizations could well have been included in Chapter 1 since it is a healthy child issue, but I wanted to give it the respect it deserves in a separate chapter. It belongs at the end of the book, however, since it is a hot issue to only a small number of people.

The overwhelming majority of my time as a pediatrician is spent reassuring parents that their children will be all right no matter what we do or don't do. It's most rewarding when I can help a child get better faster, but unfortunately that doesn't happen very often. Most of the time kids get well all by themselves. It is our job to make them feel more comfortable until they do.

Lisa Wiseman, M.D.

Acknowledgments

This book has evolved over the years from discussions I have had with parents and other caretakers. It was their demand for excellence, understanding, and participation in their children's health care that brought out the best in me, and for that I am truly appreciative. I am grateful to Dr. Mary Marvin Johnson and Dr. James Strong for giving me the opportunity to resume my career as a pediatrician after having three babies and taking a six-week maternity leave that lasted five years. Those three babies taught me in a few sleepless nights what medical school couldn't teach me in seven years.

The support of those who read the early drafts of the manuscript gave me the confidence I needed to finish the book. My mom, Dora Hauser, and my father-in-law, Dr. Charles Wiseman, each in their own way encouraged me to persevere. A special thank you is due the friends and coworkers who freely offered their support and valuable commentary. These include Anne Kane, Mary Gabel, Wanda Smith, Laura Nipp, Teri Sapp, Kimberly Currie, and Rachel Crow. Scattered pages were read by friends who called for informal advice and instead were given some homework. For this I am indebted to Julie Ligon, Anne Martin, Elizabeth Davis, Kathy Passiak, Ann Tabler, David Franklin, Jeff Honeck, and Jaye Bunde. To my other dear friends and my husband, Vince, who are so integral to my everyday routine, your presence in my life was support enough.

It is much more difficult to win the support of critical colleagues. Were it not for Dr. Joe Hanig, Dr. Debra Burns, Dr. Hope Northrup, Dr. Raquel Bono, Dr. Charles Ginsburg, and Dr. Bill Hauser I might have given up early on. When I feared the whole project would be discounted because of my nontraditional comments on nutrition, Megan Murphy, registered dietician, childhood friend, and now literary critic, barely flinched when she read the first drafts. Thanks Megan.

Until now I have been unable to express my appreciation to the mentors who have played such a role in my life. There are far too many to include all of them, but Dr. George McCracken, Dr. Daniel Levin, Dr. Wes Norman, Dr. Sherwyn Scwartz, Dr. Charles Roeth, and my high school biology and chemistry teachers, Mr. Weber and Mr. Hartman, deserve special mention. At the risk of becoming too obtuse I want to thank my typing teacher and the inventors of the personal computer (whoever they are). My English teachers had better luck with me than did my penmanship teachers. We need to pay our teachers a lot more.

This book would still be a stack of papers in a box if it weren't for the enthusiasm of Karen Berger, my publisher at QMP. I never felt luckier in my life the day Karen called and told me that she thought my sample chapters were terrific. I held my breath waiting for the "but" that never came. My editor at QMP, Carolita Deter, patiently allowed me to vent my mind and heart before skillfully nudging me in the direction she somehow knew I wanted to go. I will draw on our relationship when it comes time to parent my kids through adolescence.

Most important of all, thanks to Mom and Dad and Nannie and Pops for passing along their genes and giving me free reign to be me. They must have known all along that I would change my mind about being an airline stewardess. (I do love to fly and to tend to the needs of others, just not at the same time.)

Contents

Your Healthy Child

Nutrition

Proper nutrition is a hot topic these days, and if you keep up with all the latest, you are probably as confused as I am. I read one article recently that reported that the decreased incidence of heart disease is not the result of improved eating habits and exercise but rather the aspirin-like preservatives found in packaged foods such as Twinkies. Good news for a change!

Parents are almost as anxious about what goes into their kid's mouth as what comes out the other end. A healthy child will grow well if offered a well-balanced diet even if it seems she doesn't eat much of it.

My toddler never eats anything. What can I do to make her eat?

Nothing. Children should not be coerced to eat. It's never successful anyway and not conducive to a happy home for anyone.

How do I know if she is eating enough?

If your child is otherwise healthy and gaining weight over time, she is eating as much food as her body needs to maintain her genetically predetermined growth pattern.

She won't eat three proper meals but wants to snack all day. What can I do?

Children are naturally inclined to eat many smaller meals rather than several larger meals. Adult meal schedules are based on an 8 to 5 work schedule, not on any natural biorhythms. Eventually she will have to adapt to the real world, but if you want her to eat, it would probably help to follow her own natural schedule rather than yours.

My child won't eat any vegetables or meat. Should I worry?

Children can grow and develop well on many different diets. Look at what the children around the world eat. They don't have anywhere near the variety of foods available to us.

Sometimes my daughter eats well for a couple of weeks and then very little for a couple of months. Is that okay?

Children can get what they need to grow and stay healthy from the meals consumed over a long period of time. Growth rates are variable and inconsistent and so are eating patterns.

All my child wants is kid's cereal. Is that enough?

Iron and vitamin-fortified cereals and milk can provide all the nutrients that a child needs for growth for a long time. Try to sneak in a piece of fruit.

My kid only eats about 10 foods. Is that good enough?

Let me guess—chicken nuggets and french fries, bread, peanut butter, spaghetti, macaroni and cheese, cheese pizza, waffles, cereal, and a couple of fruits (maybe). Any child will grow well if there is an adequate supply of "fairly decent" food in the house. Keep offering "new" foods, but don't force.

Should I give her a daily vitamin?

Although it probably doesn't make any difference in a healthy child who eats a reasonable variety of foods, a multivitamin with iron supplement can be a good idea. It can keep her from getting too far behind in certain nutrients. It doesn't need to be everyday and not when she is eating relatively well. Iron is probably the most important nutrient left out in a poor diet.

Why is iron so important and why is it so hard to get enough of it?

Iron is a major component of the body's red blood cells and muscle cells. Studies have shown that children who are even mildly iron deficient perform much better on academic tests when their iron deficiency is corrected. Some nutritionists are starting to call iron-containing vitamins "smart pills." It works for my kids.

The best sources of iron are red meat, soybeans, and green leafy vegetables.

What do you think about giving "superdoses" of certain vitamins and minerals like they sell at the health food stores?

Although taking higher doses of many vitamins and minerals than the current recommended daily allowance (RDA) may have some health benefits, most of the data are still controversial and no studies have been conducted in growing children. I would hesitate to give my children anything in an amount that could not be ingested by eating a reasonable amount of food. For instance, giving a child a 500 mg vitamin C tablet is like giving him a dozen oranges to eat every day.

I think that she needs a chewable vitamin, but I've tried them all and she hates them. Any suggestions?

Food is always a good choice, but when that fails, a good multivitamin and iron-fortified kid's cereal with milk will accomplish the same thing. Many fruit juices and fruit drinks are now fortified with calcium, vitamin A, vitamin C, and other nutrients. There is even some candy disguised as "fruit snacks" that have added nutrients. Shop wisely by reading the labels.

Won't she have terrible eating habits when she grows up?

It's good to remember that children will ultimately develop the eating habits of their parents.

How much milk does she need?

Milk is formulated for rapidly growing mammals; only humans drink it long after the time for which it is intended. Many ethnic groups around the world do not drink milk after infancy and early childhood (many cannot tolerate it). If your child likes milk and continues to drink it, fine. If she does not like it or it makes her sick, don't force it. Her calcium needs can be met with other dairy products or calcium-enriched fruit juices or drinks.

Is it possible to drink too much milk?

If a child drinks milk to the exclusion of all other foods, she is likely to become deficient in iron. It would be reasonable to limit milk consumption to 24 ounces a day. If she pours it over iron-fortified cereal, then it's probably okay. Try to expose her to other foods without being a nag and be glad that milk is very nutritious.

What about fat and cholesterol?

Difficult question. Although high fat and cholesterol levels have been shown to be risk factors for heart disease and other diseases, they are just a small part of the whole picture and probably not even one of the more important parts. It is no surprise that genetics plays the biggest role. Like weight control, strict dietary manipulation of cholesterol intake has only modest effects and only over the short term.

How come? If you aren't eating any cholesterol, how can you have too much of it?

There are several reasons, but the simplest is that the liver manufactures its own cholesterol to make many molecules the body needs. Everybody has a preset genetically determined range of cholesterol levels. When dietary cholesterol is unavailable, the liver just cranks up its production.

Isn't there a medication for lowering cholesterol? Does it work?

Yes. Medications are available that "trick" the liver and interfere with its ability to manufacture cholesterol. Blood cholesterol levels drop.

Does this reduce the risk for heart disease?

It is still uncertain if this ultimately affects the incidence of heart disease. Newer information indicates that lowering the cholesterol level alone will not make any difference in the long run if other more important risk factors are present.

Should I limit my children's fat and cholesterol intake?

If there is a significant family history of early heart disease, it may be worthwhile to *reasonably* limit intake in childhood until further information is available.

Should I use 2% or skim milk?

If your child likes milk and there is a concern about future heart disease, 2% is a sensible option after the age of 2 years. Skim milk is not recommended for growing kids because they need the calories. If your child is thin and doesn't eat much solid food, but likes milk, I see no problem leaving her on whole milk.

I think my kids get plenty of fat and calories from all the french fries and chicken nuggets they eat. I'd rather they drink skim milk like my husband and me. That's okay, isn't it?

Sure. Kids whose diets are not fat restricted will do fine on skim milk. I worry about those on skim milk whose parents have them on their own restrictive dietary regimen.

What else can I do to limit fat and cholesterol in my children?

Be careful. There is flimsy evidence about the benefits of reducing fat and cholesterol in children, and there is solid evidence that doing so can affect growth. Common sense and moderation are in order.

What about sugar?

The body's major fuel is sugar (glucose to be precise). All fats, carbohydrates (sugars and starches), and proteins are converted into glucose by the body before they can be used for energy. When a cell needs glucose, it really doesn't care if it came from a potato, apple, or piece of candy.

Doesn't it have something to do with how *fast* the sugar becomes available for energy?

No. It has more to do with the fact that these other foods have additional nutrients besides sugar. The breakdown of carbohydrates into simple sugars actually begins in the mouth. The differences in energy availability are insignificant to healthy children who do not fast or run marathons.

Isn't the sugar from natural sources such as fruit better than table sugar?

Table sugar and fruit sugars are processed no differently by the body. Fruit is better than candy because fruit has additional nutrients besides sugar, but not because its sugar is "better." The overall amount of sugar consumed in a piece of fruit is less than that in a bag of candy.

Surely too much sugar is bad for you, right?

Except in diabetics, the only complication of excessive sugar intake is dental cavities, and this is rare nowadays with fluoridated water and toothpaste. The tendency for cavities is also inherited. Excessive sugar intake may indicate a poor diet overall, but if other more nutritious foods are consumed in adequate amounts, sugar just doesn't deserve all the bad publicity.

Won't too much sugar make her fat?

Ultimate adult weight is dependent on several factors, the overwhelmingly most important one being heredity. Sugar consumption plays a very small part.

What about artificial sweeteners?

I'd definitely avoid the ones known to be associated with cancer (saccharin). Moderate use of the others (aspartame) is believed to be okay. Another option is using less real sugar.

Does sugar make a child "hyper"?

Study after study has found no link between sugar consumption and a child's activity level or behavior. One interesting observation is that children get big sugar loads at birthday parties and other excitable occasions. Is it a surprise that they are a bit overexcited?

Many of the people in our family are overweight. I don't want that to happen to my child. What can I do to prevent it?

Unfortunately, not much. All scientific evidence points to weight as being strictly genetically determined. Your child's ultimate weight is not dependent on the dietary habits he has as a child.

Are you telling me it doesn't matter what I do and I should just give up?

No. It is important to cultivate good eating and exercise habits in your child for many other reasons besides ultimate adult weight. I am saying that you cannot alter his genetic predisposition to be overweight or not.

How can she become fat if I limit her calories?

You may be able to limit her caloric intake when she is very young and keep her thinner than she otherwise would be for a while. Eventually though, as she controls her own eating habits, her genetic predisposition will manifest itself. Try to teach her what's best, even if she doesn't always do it.

Wouldn't keeping her thin as a child help her to stay thinner and eat right in the long run?

Scientific evidence has repeatedly demonstrated that weight loss due to strict dietary control is not sustainable. I would be more worried about the psychological effects on a young child whose mother thinks her weight is that important. Building her self-esteem is more worthy of your efforts. I would be more concerned about what goes into my child's head than what goes into her mouth!

I don't like the sound of this. I know it's not good for her to be overweight. As her mother, shouldn't I be doing something about it?

Set a good example. Be supportive and teach her about the many benefits of good food and exercise. As your child gets older, weight control may become important to *her*. She may try to regulate her weight with diet and exercise routines and under these circumstances is more likely to be successful. Eating good, healthy food and participating in athletics have many rewards, only one of which is weight management.

If she fanatically watches her diet and exercises daily, she'll be thin, right?

The results of her efforts will be a reflection of who and what she is. Even with the very best support and effort, successful weight control is modest and relatively short lived overall (look at Oprah), but feeling good about oneself can last a lifetime. Remember that your child's ultimate weight and eating and exercise habits will be a reflection of your own.

What happened to the four basic food groups? I don't like this pyramid thing.
I don't know. Me either.

Growth, Growth Charts, and Growing Pains

Children really do grow in spurts rather than at a steady pace. They grow at their own individual genetically determined rates, and unless a child is not fed or lives in an otherwise hostile environment, he will grow on his own schedule.

What do you mean by individual "genetically determined rate"?
Genes inherited in various combinations from previous generations determine a person's ultimate height and weight. The *timetable* for growth is also inherited. For example, in some families the children are "runts" through grade school and then grow dramatically in their late teens to become large adults. In other families children reach their adult size by the sixth grade and then scarcely grow at all after that.

How do I know if my child is growing normally?
Most physicians weigh patients and measure their height at regular intervals and plot them on growth charts. As long as your child is headed in the right direction, she's doing okay.

It seems that she doesn't grow at all for the longest time and then she shoots up over the weekend. Am I imaging this?
No. Kids do grow in well-defined spurts. They don't grow at a constant pace as the pink and blue growth charts imply.

My son was in the 95th percentile when he was born and has been there for the past 9 months. Is he going to be big enough for pro football?
I wouldn't count on it. The growth charts were prepared prior to 1950 using the statistics on infants born in Denver, Colorado. The charts are out of date. Nowadays, babies are born bigger, are more likely to be formula fed, experience less childhood illness, etc. The charts are still valid for demonstrating overall trends, but the absolute numbers are not meaningful anymore. Most babies are born well above the 50th percentile now. I've

heard rumors that the growth charts are being revised to reflect current statistics.

We're from Taiwan, but our baby was born in the United States. Will he be a lot taller growing up in a healthier environment and having a better diet?

Not likely. Unless your family is small because of inadequate nutrition or illness, your baby will be approximately the same size as other family members born in Taiwan.

My daughter was in the 90th percentile; for the last 6 months her growth has slowed and now she is in the 50th percentile. Should I be worried?

Probably not. Babies are born bigger now than they used to be. As they get older, their growth adjusts according to their genetic predisposition. Unless she comes from a really tall family, she was going to slow down eventually.

Why are babies bigger than they used to be?

Mostly because their moms are healthier. They have their first babies at an older age, a greater time elapses between pregnancies, and they have fewer babies overall. They smoke and drink less, have better diets, and are in better physical shape. They take prenatal vitamins and get good prenatal medical care.

Overall, aren't children bigger than they used to be?

Yes. Maternal factors account for the larger size of newborns and young infants, but improved nutrition and fewer childhood illnesses account for the trend toward larger toddlers. When these kids grow up, their children may be larger still since they will have even healthier parents.

What are "growing pains"?

Healthy children frequently complain of foot and leg pain at night intermittently throughout the early childhood years. "Growing pains" is just a descriptive term for this common complaint when no other physical abnormalities can be found. It may or may not be related to growth at all.

What causes them?

No one knows why kids get growing pains. It's most common during periods of increased physical exertion, but that's not always the case. Since children have been known to grow half an inch overnight, some discomfort at the end of a long, active day is not surprising.

How bad are these pains?

Most growing pains are mild and are only mentioned to the pediatrician incidentally during routine checkups. Rarely they can be so frequent and severe that blood tests or x-rays are ordered to rule out serious pathology.

What can I do when my son hurts so much he wakes at night, cries, and can't go back to sleep?

Tender loving care and gentle massage are usually all that's needed. Occasionally you might need to try some Tylenol or Motrin.

Developmental Skills

Acquiring developmental skills is highly variable and individual. Unless a child lives in a hostile environment he will progress at his own pace. Nothing will speed it along. When a child is making rapid progress in one area, usually other areas slow down or even regress a bit. Early walkers may be late talkers or vice versa.

This is my first baby and I've read all the books. She's ahead of schedule in some things and lagging behind in others. Should I be concerned?

Probably not. Unless she is not making any progress in a specific area or very little progress in several areas over time, there is no cause for concern.

My son sat up and crawled *early*, but he's 14 months old now and still not walking. Is this abnormal?

No. A child will sit, crawl, walk, and talk when he's ready. Children who walk at 9 months are not any better at it in the long run (no pun intended) than those who don't walk until they are 15 months.

My son is almost 2 years old and says only a few words. My doctor isn't worried because he says he has "language." What does that mean?

If he says a few words appropriately he can talk, and if he communicates his needs and wants even without actual speech, he has "language." Late talkers may start with full sentences rather than single syllables.

Is it too early to "potty train" my 18-month-old?

It may take 12 months to completely train an 18-month-old; it takes a couple of weeks to successfully train a 3½-year-old. It's so much easier if you (or even better, your child) picks the right time. Some parents have successfully trained their 18-month-olds, but at what price? What would she have been doing during the time that she was concentrating on the toilet?

My 3-year-old is very bright and is learning to read at his Montessori school. What else should I be doing to help him succeed?

If your child is bright and is in a nurturing environment, he will succeed. Let him pick and choose what he wants to do because that is more likely to coincide with where he is developmentally than what you want him to do. You may want him to read, but he may be working on gross motor skills and wants to jump and climb.

Isn't it better to get an early start?

What a 3-year-old can be painstakingly taught in 6 months, a 6-year-old can pick up on his own in a week. That sure frees up a lot of time that can be spent on more age-appropriate activities (i.e., "playing").

My daughter is really bright and needs a lot of mentally stimulating activities. What do you recommend?

Bright children are terrific at enriching and entertaining themselves and don't need anyone to do so for them. "Keeping her occupied" may actually be a disservice to a child whose own mind is full of ideas.

I don't want her to get bored. Shouldn't I sign her up for some lessons or something?

Before signing her up, think carefully about what she would be doing otherwise. If the answer is watching TV, sign her up. She probably needs a more nurturing environment.

I know she watches too much TV, but we only fight when I turn it off. How can I encourage her to do other things?

What do you do in *your* free time? Set a good example. A family that participates in a lot of different activities will have children that have a lot better things to do than watch TV.

I don't want to be pushy, but all the other kids are doing so many things. Won't my son get left behind?

Not necessarily. Life has become very competitive and there is pressure to make your kids excel and stand out early. It's just big business to get young kids involved early in as much as possible. There's more interest in your wallet than your child. Just because someone is willing to take your money and "teach" your kids something doesn't mean it is the best thing to do for your child. Earlier is not necessarily better. I'd rather my kids succeed later when it really matters than peak when they are 8 or 18 years.

What if he wants to do something I just can't do or know nothing about?

It's rare to hear about all the wonderful lessons that successful musicians, artists, athletes, and intellectuals had as a child. It's more common to hear about their difficult childhoods and all the other obstacles they had to overcome. It's not the lessons or teachers that make the difference, it's the child. Children will pursue the activities that they find rewarding. Relax, you'll know when it's time for lessons.

My 8-year-old daughter is an excellent gymnast with world-class potential. How can I give her a well-balanced life?

This is a really tough question, but here's what I think: To be world class at anything you have to be world class in many things. Everything has to come together exactly right and for a long time without significant interruption (e.g., talent, single-minded dedication, self-motivation, lots of being in the right place at the right time, and proper body type now and later with no injuries, illnesses, or accidents).

It also takes time and money and the cooperation and single-minded dedication of everyone else in the family. The talent and dedication may be a sure thing, but everything else can change in a heartbeat. If your child is only 8 years old, there are many years during which things can go wrong. What then? Patch her up and send her out again and again? Each time you do this the investment becomes larger and the eventual loss that much greater.

It is a difficult choice. If your daughter has what it takes and wants to pursue her goal, there are many things to be gained (and lost) along the way. Don't stand in her way. World-class athletes wouldn't be diverted. But if she starts to falter, be supportive and let her decide no matter what investment you have already made.

Genetics and Heredity

All living things are products of their genes. The newspapers are filled daily with new reports of yet another trait or tendency that is inherited and on which chromosome it is located. The nature vs. nurture argument rages on, and although unpopular and "politically incorrect" to say so, the nature corner is winning.

How do scientists differentiate the effects of environment and genetics and come to all these conclusions?

Mostly they study identical twins reared apart and children who were not reared by their biologic parents.

And what do they find?

Their findings indicate that children become more like their biologic parents as time goes by regardless of the varied environments in which they are raised.

How can they discount the effect of the environment so easily?

They don't. Environment is very important, but it is just another expression of a person's genetic makeup. People create their environments according to their own genetic predispositions.

How do they know it's not the other way around, that is, that the environment creates the person?

Children not only inherit their parents' genes but they also grow up in an environment of their parents' making. For instance, intellectuals buy books (and often are attracted to and marry other intellectuals) and musicians buy instruments (and often are attracted to and marry other musicians). Their children will inherit their intellectual and musical talents and grow up in houses surrounded by books and music, respectively. The child's environment is just another "dose" of the parents' genes.

If genetics is so important, how come children aren't more exact copies of their parents?

Even though genes are very powerful, the way they are copied and mutated and divided and distributed before being passed on to the next generation is quite complex. Every individual is unique and unpredictable, but there's usually a strong family resemblance.

My son has asthma and my doctor said it's inherited. There's no family history of asthma as far as anyone can remember. Is that possible?

Yes. It is not necessary for anyone else in the family to have a disease that is inherited. There are several reasons for this. First of all, spontaneous mutations do occur. Second, but much more important, there is variability in the expression of inherited conditions. What this means is that it's possible that there are other manifestations of allergic disease in your family that are not recognized as such, for example, sensitive skin, hay fever, or bronchitis. Third, Americans in general tend to have very small families, and even if a condition has a very strong hereditary component, you may not see it for generations if the families are small.

It sounds like "genetics rules" and there's not much I can do about it. Isn't that depressing?

Pessimism must run in your family. I think just the opposite. It takes the pressure off. I am what I am and so are my children.

Miscellaneous Health Questions

My child is now 6 years old and in school. He has had all his immunizations. Does he still need a checkup every year?

I'm sure that if you had any concerns about your child's growth or development or any underlying illnesses or problems you wouldn't be asking. The answer is no. It would be extremely unlikely to pick up any significant health problems on a routine checkup. School-age kids are brought to the pediatrician periodically for illnesses, and you can stay informed about any new immunizations or screening tests that he may need during those visits. He can be weighed and measured and have his blood pressure checked then also. Of course, if you ever have any concerns or questions about your child's health, you should not wait until the annual checkup anyway.

How often does my child need a urinalysis or blood count?

A routine blood count is performed late in the first year of life when anemia is most likely to appear. Unless you or your doctor has some reason to suspect anemia, a routine blood count is not necessary. Screening urinalysis is no longer recommended in healthy children who do not have any personal or family history of urinary problems.

What about a lead screen?

The most recent data have indicated that the percentage of children found to have toxic levels of lead in their blood has dropped dramatically since the last studies were done in the late seventies and early eighties. It went from around 90% to less than 10%. However, the percentage in poor, black, inner-city children is 35%. Universal screening is still controversial. Most pediatricians order screens on an individual basis.

What about a TB test?

The recommendations on this are changing, although most schools still require them. Screening for tuberculosis is only useful in high-risk populations; the screening of schoolchildren during the past several decades was not justified. It is doubtful, however, that this will change anytime soon since there is now an increasing number of TB cases, mostly because of AIDS and immigration.

Does my child need a camp or sports physical?

This is more of a liability issue than a medical one. Routine physicals in healthy children who receive regular medical care are not productive, but the camp or coach has no way of knowing which children get regular medical care and which ones don't. I think that a signed statement by the physician allowing participation should be satisfactory. Let the physician decide if a particular child needs to be examined or not. This would save the insurance companies money and parents, children, and doctors a lot of time.

2

Getting Down to Basics

How Sick Is Sick?

The first question I ask a mom when she brings her child into the office is, "Is she sick?" The indignant mom is probably thinking, "Why else would I bring her in?"

Every time I call my pediatrician's office for an appointment, the nurse asks me if my daughter is sick or not. It really makes me mad! How sick does she have to be to get an appointment?

The nurse is trying to decide if your child needs to be seen immediately or not. If a child is really "sick," she needs to be seen as soon as possible.

When is a child "sick"?

A "sick" child is one whose protective defense mechanisms (coughing, sneezing, runny nose, swollen glands and sore throat, fever, congestion, vomiting, and diarrhea) are not successfully warding off microbial invasion. Rather than an improvement in these typical symptoms after a few days, a "sick" child deteriorates.

But wouldn't she get better sooner if I brought her in right away so the pediatrician could "nip it in the bud"?

No. Her own body is much better at keeping her from getting sick than any medication. What a parent perceives as illness, the coughing, sneezing, runny nose, fever, swollen glands and sore throat, congestion, vomiting, or diarrhea, the pediatrician views as *normal physiologic mechanisms* for defending the body. Although many medications try to blunt the body's defenses, they are not very good at it. They also have a lot of side effects that may be worse than the symptoms they are trying unsuccessfully to treat.

So you're saying it's okay that she has all these symptoms that are making her feel so bad?

Not only okay but necessary. A child develops immunity with each new challenge. The more battles fought as a child, the fewer battles she will have to fight as an adult.

Is it reasonable then to just keep an eye on her at home for a few days?

If you feel comfortable that her symptoms are typical of routine childhood illness, then, sure, watch her for a few days and most likely she will improve all on her own.

How do I know that her symptoms are typical of a routine childhood illness?

After you've been through it a few times.

What if I am just not sure?

That's when the pediatrician can help, usually with just a phone call. Most of a pediatrician's time is spent reassuring moms that everything is going to be okay.

Is there anything specifically that I should watch out for?

Rather than looking for danger signs, it is easier and more helpful to look for good signs. A child who is interested in her environment, is easily consoled, takes fluids, and has occasional periods of playfulness is doing fine. A child who is well enough to whine and fuss until she gets what she wants is doing great!

What if some of her symptoms seem particularly severe or she is having pain?

That's another reason for having a pediatrician. Most likely you will just get another dose of reassurance, but sometimes medication can make a difference even if only temporarily. It is rare that pediatricians actually get to take credit for curing anybody.

How do you know when medication may help?

It is usually fairly easy to make a diagnosis and decide what treatment is needed by listening to the mom describe the child's symptoms and by performing a careful physical examination.

Sometimes the pediatrician still doesn't know what's wrong, then what?

This happens frequently. If the child is not really sick, it is better to wait and see what will happen in the next day or so. Almost always there are signs of improvement. If a child appears to be really "sick," then blood tests, x-rays, or cultures are helpful. Pediatricians love to order tests and prescribe medications. That is why most of us went to medical school. We just don't get to do so that often.

My pediatrician always has me bring my child in but never does anything? What's the point?

Doing nothing is doing something.

Temperature/Fever, Brain Damage, and Convulsions

Body temperature cycles naturally over a range of about 2 degrees in a 24-hour period. It is lowest early in the morning and highest late in the afternoon. Children have a wider fluctuation in body temperature than adults, and "normal" may range from about 97° to 100° F. Although the average body temperature is approximately 98.6° F, it is seldom at this exact reading.

There are many misconceptions about fever in children. Let's go down the list of some of the most common ones.

1. "The higher the fever, the more serious the illness." *Not.* Generally speaking, children with self-limiting viral infections tend to have higher temperatures than those with potentially more dangerous bacterial infections. In addition, low-grade fevers (99° to 100° F) do not necessarily mean that the illness is any less serious.

2. "When you take the temperature under the armpit, you add a degree; in the rectum, you subtract a degree; and under the tongue, it's just right." *It doesn't matter!* Body temperatures fluctuate widely during illness and there may be a difference of 1 to 2 degrees in relatively short periods of time. Adding or subtracting that degree really doesn't tell you anything useful.

3. "Fever is the best way to determine how sick your child is." *Also not true.* Very sick kids can have normal body temperatures and healthy kids can have very high body temperatures. Fever is just one of the many factors considered when determining the seriousness of an illness.

4. "Get the fever down anyway you can." *Not true.* Fever is protective, and treatment is unnecessary unless the child is clearly miserable because of the fever itself (and not the illness in general).
5. "High fevers can cause convulsions." *Not exactly.* A certain percentage of the population (around 4% or so) will experience a so-called febrile seizure in the first year or two of life. How high the fever is doesn't have anything to do with it. In predisposed children a low-grade temperature is just as likely to elicit a seizure as a higher one.
6. "High fevers cause brain damage." *Not true.* The brain actually signals the body to raise the temperature to kill germs, not the other way around. This is work (the heart rate, blood pressure, and respiratory rate increase), and before the process becomes too stressful or can cause any harm, the brain signals the body to lower the temperature for a while so the child can rest. (Incidentally, fever-reducing medications interfere with the brain's signal.) After a brief respite, up it goes again, and the cycle continues until all the germs are destroyed and the child recovers.

What is fever?

Fever is a mechanism for protecting the body from foreign invaders such as viruses or bacteria. Germs invade humans (as opposed to other living organisms) because they survive best in an environment of around 98.6° F. The human body fights back by raising body temperatures to levels that kill the invaders. Most of our infection-fighting cells and their chemical weapons work better at higher temperatures. In addition to killing the germs, an elevated temperature is also an early sign of impending illness and its resolution usually signals that the illness is beginning to subside. Fever is actually our friend not our foe.

I hear those new ear thermometers are exact to the tenth of a degree?

Yeah, but so what?

If body temperature fluctuates so widely, how do I know if my baby has a fever or not?

A good rule of thumb is that any single reading over 100 degrees (no matter where it is taken) means fever is present. There is usually no need to repeatedly take the child's temperature unless his condition deteriorates several days later when you would expect him to be recovering. If several readings are under 100° F in the first couple of days of an illness, there is probably no fever associated with this particular illness.

Why does fever seem to "come and go"?

It is normal for body temperature to fluctuate. If you get a reading of around 98° F or so, that doesn't mean the fever is gone. Most likely it will go up again and down again many times in the first few days of an illness before it goes down and stays down.

How long should a fever typically last?

A fever is almost always gone by the third or fourth day of an illness. Many don't even last that long. If it goes away only to return a day or two later, it can signal a complication and you should talk to your doctor.

My child has a temperature of 104° F and you say he's not even sick! What do you mean?

Frequently a child with a very high fever does not even appear ill. What this means is that he is effectively using his infection-fighting mechanisms. I see this most commonly in children with throat viruses.

If what you say is true, why should I even bother to take my child's temperature?

Good question. Most parents know when their child is sick and don't need a thermometer to tell them what they already know, regardless if there is a fever or not.

Should I throw away the thermometer?

I wouldn't go that far. A child's body temperature can be a useful piece of the puzzle. A thermometer is helpful to less experienced caretakers (school personnel and babysitters), and it can get the doctor's attention in the middle of the night.

I'm a new mom and I can't tell if my newborn is sick or not. Shouldn't I take his temperature?

Yes. Babies under 2 months of age can be very tricky and do not show predictable signs of illness. If you think your newborn might be sick, call the doctor regardless of the temperature (see Chapter 4). One of the factors the pediatrician will consider is the infant's temperature.

My baby feels so bad! Will it hurt to give her some Tylenol?

No. Lowering the fever artificially with acetaminophen (Tylenol) or ibuprofen (Motrin or Advil) probably won't make much of a difference in her eventual recovery, but it may make her feel a little better temporarily. Go ahead as long as she cooperates. I don't recommend holding her down, prying her jaws apart, and shoving bad-tasting medicine down her throat. She feels bad enough already!

What about a cool or tepid bath?
This is generally not a good idea unless she truly enjoys a tepid bath and you are careful to prevent any shivering. When body temperature drops too quickly, reflexive muscular action induces shivering and that actually elevates the temperature.

Should I take all her clothes off?
Only if she likes to be naked.

What about a cold cloth on the forehead?
It might make you feel better.

Alcohol sponge bath?
Why? Fever is good, remember? Alcohol is not.

So what should I do?
You don't *have* to do anything, but babies might like sucking on a clean washcloth that has been dipped in cool or even cold water. Many of the highest fevers are caused by viral throat infections, and this not only may soothe some of the discomfort but provides a little fluid as well. Toddlers and older kids do great with popsicles, ice cream, and ice-cold drinks.

I've done all that and she is still burning up. Now what?
The goal is to increase the child's comfort, not to decrease the child's body temperature.

Can giving Tylenol right away prevent a febrile seizure?
No. These seizures almost always occur very early in the illness (usually when the temperature shoots up quickly the first time) before anyone knows the child is even sick yet. For this reason, seizures cannot be prevented with fever-reducing medications.

My son had a "febrile seizure" on the third day of his illness? Could it have been prevented with Tylenol?
Extremely unlikely. Occasionally a febrile seizure occurs 2 to 3 days into an illness. If this has happened to your child, it is reasonable to treat the febrile illnesses more aggressively from the start. More likely, though, a seizure that occurs 2 to 3 days into an illness is due to the illness itself, not the fever per se.

I always worry about convulsions when my child has a fever. Are you saying I shouldn't?

No, you shouldn't. Although febrile seizures can be very scary and frequently result in a trip to the emergency department and occasionally hospitalization, they have no short- or long-term significance beyond their ability to elicit panic.

How high does the fever have to be to cause a seizure?

Children who tend to get febrile seizures can develop them even if their body temperatures are normal. Children who don't, don't get them even at temperatures above 105° F.

If a child is prone to febrile seizures, will it happen every time a fever occurs?

No. Usually they only get one or two episodes altogether before they outgrow them.

How come it's called a febrile seizure? It seems that the fever isn't really related to the seizure at all?

You're right. There's a good chance that the fever itself is not responsible for febrile seizures. More likely the virus that elicits the fever also triggers the seizure (i.e., the seizure is just a part of the illness).

Can viruses do this?

Yes. Herpesviruses and others are very likely responsible for many febrile seizures. This explains why the seizures can accompany a low-grade fever, why they develop early in the illness even if the fever lasts for several days, and why they don't occur every time there is a fever even if it is very high. It would also explain why most kids have only one or sometimes two before they outgrow them and also why there are no short-term or long-term consequences.

How so?

Only a limited number of viruses can cause seizures in early childhood. Most kids never get more than a couple of these viral infections.

How high can I let a fever go before I need to do something?

What are you planning to do? If you and your doctor are confident that your child has a routine illness, there's nothing you should do other than make your child as comfortable as possible until he recovers on his own.

Contagiousness

Contagiousness is a subject of much concern these days since so many young children (who get sick more often) are in some sort of day care setting.

Certain generalizations apply to contagiousness. These are the guidelines I use in my office.

1. Viruses, which are responsible for most colds (upper respiratory infections), pinkeye, sore throats, flu, and many rashes, are spread fairly easily to anyone who hasn't already had them and who comes into direct contact with infectious mucous secretions. The virus is concentrated in the mucus and infects others when it gets on a child's hands and then on everything he touches.

2. Viruses that are responsible for vomiting, diarrhea, and stomach flu are concentrated in the stools and vomitus. The bathroom is quickly contaminated with virus, and once on your hands, the virus can easily be spread throughout the house. If contaminated hands come in contact with the mouth, a person can become infected. Unlike nasal discharge, however, diarrhea and vomiting are intermittent and so easier to confine to a single bathroom that can be disinfected after each use. Combined with good handwashing, this can limit the spread of gastrointestinal illness to other family members.

3. Rashes are usually manifestations of upper respiratory or gastrointestinal illnesses and the same guidelines apply to these kinds of viruses.

4. A fever usually indicates that the child is contagious. If there are enough viral particles around to elicit fever, there are probably enough to infect others. Fever is a reasonable approximation of contagiousness when present, but absence of fever does not mean that the child is not contagious.

5. If an infection is caused by bacteria and is treated with antibiotics, the child is considered contagious for 12 to 24 hours after the medication is begun. Bacteria that cause infections of the ears, nose, throat, skin, lungs, and sinuses are not easily passed to others; in fact, they are very difficult to pass along even to family members. Children usually "catch" these infections after contracting a viral illness that has weakened them and because of their unique anatomy. Children with diarrhea caused by bacteria should be considered contagious for as long as they have diarrhea, even if they have been on antibiotics for more than 12 to 24 hours.

How do you know if an illness is contagious or not?

By definition all infectious diseases are contagious. However, the degree, the duration, and the mechanism of contagiousness can vary widely depending on the type of germ, even among very close germ relatives.

How do you know how long a child is contagious?

There are innumerable viruses, dozens of bacteria, and a smattering of other microbes and parasites that infect children, each with its own unique timetable for spreadability. Some are well known, but most are not, and it's just an educated guess when it's "safe to go back in the water" so to speak.

In our family we are very careful about not eating and drinking after each other. My kids always use a tissue and cover their mouths when they cough or sneeze. How come we still pass around all our colds?

Although I would not recommend drinking or eating after someone with a cold or sore throat and I would avoid the sneezes and coughs of others, handwashing is a much more important way to avoid infection. It would be better to sneeze and cough down toward your feet instead of onto your hands.

As a pediatrician, I've trained myself to wash my hands compulsively and to avoid touching my face. Germs can survive for many hours in mucus that has dried on hands or tissues (or toys or doorknobs or sleeves). Most families cannot avoid passing around these kinds of viruses, especially to the other children in the household. Parents might be able to if they avoid touching their own faces and wash their hands frequently.

If the viruses that cause upper respiratory infections are so easily spread, why doesn't everyone in the house come down with them?

Generally speaking, you can't get the exact same virus more than once. As you get older, it is more likely you've already had a particular virus and have become immune. There are hundreds of viruses. Have you noticed that older people don't get as many colds?

I've noticed that my kids always get sick when they are worn out. Why is that?

The body carries on many important tasks simultaneously and not all functions can operate at peak levels all the time. Fighting infection is just one of these functions, and sometimes the immune system has to take a backseat so other more crucial functions can work at peak efficiency.

Adults feel "stressed out" when expected to do more than they feel comfortably able to do. The body works double time to keep up, and there's just not much reserve left for fighting infection. If a person comes into contact with a pathogenic microbe at this time, he is much more likely to get sick. This is true of children to some extent, but mostly they get sick often because they are constantly coming into contact with germs that they've never encountered before.

How long is a cold contagious?

Colds (upper respiratory infections) are probably contagious for the first several days. Once a child has "turned the corner" and seems to be improving, it is unlikely that the virus will spread to others. Since there are so many different viruses that cause colds, it is impossible to be more specific than that.

How long is a child with vomiting and diarrhea contagious?

As long as the vomiting and diarrhea continue.

Once the fever is gone, a child is no longer contagious, right?

Wrong. The absence of fever does *not* mean that the person is not contagious. Early in an infection before the body has had time to mount a febrile response, there is frequently enough virus present to infect others and the child may not even feel sick yet.

A good example is chickenpox. Children are most contagious a couple of days before the first spot or fever appears. Fever may persist later in the illness, although not enough virus is left to infect others.

When can my child go back to school?

When (1) she feels well enough to stay all day and participate in normal activities, (2) her fever is gone, (3) symptoms are clearly improving, (4) prescribed medications have been taken for at least 12 hours, and (5) vomiting and diarrhea are gone.

What if she still has a rash?

If all the above criteria are met, she can return to school in most instances even if she still has a rash.

3

The Medicine Cabinet

Medications for Reducing Fever and Pain

ASPIRIN

Aspirin is the gold standard by which all medications for reducing fever and pain are compared. However, because of its rare but potentially fatal association with a disease known as Reye's syndrome, no child should ever be given aspirin for routine fever or pain control. Your doctor may still prescribe it for some uncommon childhood conditions. Overdoses can be toxic and aspirin should always be kept out of the reach of children and teenagers.

ACETAMINOPHEN

Historically, acetaminophen has been considered a safe and effective drug for reducing fever. It comes in many concentrations and flavors and is available as a liquid, pill, chewable tablet, and suppository. Although rectal absorption is variable, an acetaminophen suppository may be the only way to medicate a vomiting or uncooperative child. For these reasons, acetaminophen is the drug of choice for reducing fever in children. However, it has no anti-inflammatory properties and is not always the best choice for controlling pain.

Just what is inflammation anyway? I thought it meant swelling.

Inflammation is the process in which the body heals itself. Blood is sent to the site of injury to deliver chemicals that cleanse the area, kill the germs, and initiate repairs. This results in swelling, redness, warmth, drainage, and tenderness at the injured site (whether a broken bone or cold in the nose). Patients whose inflammatory responses are blunted due to medication or other underlying medical conditions do not heal well and are at risk for serious complications after even minor insults.

Even though most childhood complaints of pain or discomfort involve some degree of inflammation, most children can be made comfortable with acetaminophen, which leaves their protective inflammatory responses intact.

IBUPROFEN

If the pain is more severe and cannot be controlled by acetaminophen (Tylenol for short) or if there is a marked inflammatory response, ibuprofen (Motrin for short) may be the best choice, especially in the first 24 to 48 hours. Unlike Tylenol, it blunts the inflammatory response, which is why it is more effective for relieving pain or discomfort. Motrin is also available in many forms and has the additional advantage of exerting its effects for 6 to 8 hours as opposed to 3 to 4 hours for Tylenol.

Motrin is a newer drug than Tylenol and there is not as much experience with frequent or intermittent long-term use in children. Because of this, I try to limit its use to the first 24 to 48 hours of an illness when the discomfort is most severe. Beyond that, Tylenol usually provides sufficient relief. I prefer Motrin over Tylenol for sore throats, sinusitis, and ear infections, which tend to be more painful, and for bone, muscle, or joint injuries, which tend to cause marked inflammation.

Why would you use a pain reliever that may interfere with healing?

Even though Motrin may retard the healing process a bit, it is usually of no clinical significance. Also, patients in pain do not heal as well as patients whose pain is controlled, so it's a trade-off.

Should I alternate between Tylenol and Motrin?

The manufacturer's package insert specifically advises against alternating acetaminophen and ibuprofen, although nurses and physicians commonly recommend this for fever control when parents phone for advice. Clinical tests have not been performed to provide evidence that this is helpful or harmful.

Then which one should I use?

If your child is ill, Tylenol is the better choice unless there is considerable discomfort or pain or excessive inflammation. Fever does not need to be "controlled" at all, but medication can make a child more comfortable. At bedtime a dose of Motrin may increase the likelihood of everyone getting a good night's sleep. If your child is not ill but rather has a sprained ankle, Motrin is the better choice.

It seems to me that Motrin works better and lasts longer. Why shouldn't I just use it whenever my son has fever or pain?

Motrin has the potential to cause serious kidney damage in patients who are dehydrated. When children are sick, they often have fever, do not drink fluids well, vomit or have diarrhea, and breathe rapidly, all of which contribute to dehydration. Almost by definition sick kids start dehydrating. Now that Motrin is available over the counter, I worry that kidney problems in children are going to increase from the frequent, casual use of ibuprofen.

Medications for Allergies and Colds

ANTIHISTAMINES

Antihistamines are some of the most commonly used drugs in children. They are most effective for conditions in which histamine is released into tissues. Antihistamines are found in many over-the-counter cold, allergy, and cough medications and also in some skin creams used for itchy rashes or insect bites.

What is histamine?

Histamine is one of many chemicals released by cells as a defense against intruders or perceived intruders in the case of allergies. In an effort to prevent an offensive agent from entering the body, histamine causes blood vessels to dilate ("congestion"), causes smooth muscle cells to contract, and provokes itching.

What are antihistamines?

Antihistamines counteract the effects of histamine. There are two basic types, sedating and nonsedating. The more familiar sedating antihistamines are Benadryl (diphenhydramine), Chlor-Trimeton (chlorpheniramine), and Dimetane (brompheniramine). They are as effective as the newer antihistamines available only by prescription. One of these is almost always found in cold, allergy, and cough medicines unless they say "nondrowsy" on the box.

In addition to their antihistamine effects, these drugs are good cough suppressants and sleeping pills. They have been around for a long time and are safe, cheap, and widely available over the counter. However, bothersome side effects include dry mouth, constipation, and urinary retention.

The widely promoted newer nonsedating antihistamines include Seldane, Hismanal, Claritin, Tavist, Allegra, and Zyrtec. They are no more effective than the time-honored antihistamines but have the advantages of having fewer side effects and being less sedating and longer lasting. You can take one in the morning and be alert all day and not need another one for 12 to 24 hours or even several days in the case of Hismanal.

If all the antihistamines are equally effective, which should I choose for my children?

It usually depends on a child's age. An older child doesn't want to feel drowsy or take medication while at school. The newer prescription antihistamines would be a better choice. On the other hand, a preschooler can be dosed with a sedating medication as needed during the day. Most mothers will be grateful for the drowsiness it produces. Preschoolers are not usually bothered by the common side effects. If an older child can tolerate the "fuzzy-headed" feeling caused by the sedating antihistamines, taking one at night might help him sleep. Not all the newer antihistamines are approved for children of all ages. Check the label.

How come Benadryl makes my child wild, not sleepy!

About 10% of children will react this way to some antihistamines. They are just wired differently, but that does not mean that your child will react that way to all antihistamines. Try a different one.

Is it okay to take both kinds of antihistamines on the same day?

Although these medications (with the exception of Seldane) are very safe, you should talk to your doctor. The occasional use of more than one type is usually okay as long as you know which ones wear off quickly and which ones last a long time. Antihistamines work best when a steady level of medication is maintained, but only children with the most severe allergies or asthma take antihistamines regularly enough to achieve that.

I want to give my child a prescription antihistamine, but he won't swallow a pill. What can I do?

Some antihistamines are now available in liquid form.

My children have a lot of runny noses and congestion, and I give them antihistamines all the time. How come they don't work that well?

There may be a couple of reasons for this. First of all, an antihistamine can lose its effects after frequent long-term use. Switching to a different antihistamine may help. Another reason is that histamine is just one of the many body substances that can cause a runny nose and congestion. For example, a runny nose and congestion due to a cold virus are not the result of histamine release. You can expect some degree of relief for a runny nose caused by an allergy but not one that is caused by a cold virus. Sometimes it is difficult to tell the difference, and many people with colds also have allergies and vice versa.

What if you can't tell if it's a cold or allergy?

My best advice is to try giving your child some Benadryl if you suspect an allergic component or if there is a strong family history of allergy. If she gets any relief and is not bothered by drowsiness, hyperactivity, or dry mouth, then use it as needed. If it seems to be just a cold, I wouldn't recommend antihistamine unless the cough is so frequent the child cannot sleep. In this case, I would use Benadryl at naptime and bedtime and give plenty of fluids to keep secretions loose. (This, of course, won't work if the child is one of those 10% that Benadryl makes hyper, but you probably already knew that.)

My child has asthma and my doctor and the label say not to give antihistamines to asthmatics. Is that right?

Asthmatics were once told to avoid antihistamines since they cause smooth muscle contraction and can make bronchial constriction worse. It was also believed that they may make lung mucus too thick to cough up because of their drying effects. This is all theoretically true. Since asthma is an allergic disease and there are now good bronchodilating drugs such as albuterol (Ventolin and Proventil) available, it is now thought that the antiallergic effects of antihistamines can benefit these patients if they also take bronchodilating medications and drink plenty of fluids.

I use Caladryl lotion for my child's itchy rashes. It's a mess. Is it worth it?

The itching caused by many rashes, especially allergic ones such as dermatitis, poison ivy, hives, and insect bites, can be reduced with oral or topical antihistamines. They even help the itch from chickenpox. It's pretty hard to overdose, but don't use both oral and topical medications. Pick the most convenient one, which usually depends on the extent of the rash. Remember other substances besides histamine may be contributing to the itch.

DECONGESTANTS

If you read labels, you will find that these potent stimulants (pseudo-ephedrine, phenylpropanolamine, and phenylephrine) are the main ingredients of most cold formulas. The purpose of decongestants is to shrink dilated blood vessels in the nose (caused by colds or allergies) and make it easier for your child to breathe. The biggest problem with these drugs is that the large dose needed to get significant nasal relief is often intolerable to the rest of the child.

Decongestants don't just constrict blood vessels in the nose, but in the entire body. Although not a problem in most children, they increase blood pressure. They are also powerful cardiac and central nervous system stimulants. Children get stomachaches and headaches, become hyperactive and jittery, and can't eat, sleep, or urinate. This is a classic example of a medication being much worse than the condition you are trying to treat, and it's waiting at a grocery store near you! I rarely recommend oral decongestants and never in infants.

My baby is so stopped up she can't breathe. What can I do?

Unfortunately, not much, but rest assured that she can breathe well enough through her mouth. Sneezing, coughing, and vomiting are nature's way of clearing secretions so she can breathe. You may be able to help her out a little by using the bulb syringe or a tissue, but she's going to feel bad for a couple of days no matter what.

I hate for my son to miss school just for a cold. He doesn't feel that bad, it's just that he's so stopped up he's uncomfortable. Will a decongestant help?

What does work well when used with caution are *topical* decongestants, specifically Afrin (oxymetazoline). In children who are at least 6 years or so, a "little" spray into one or both nostrils lasts 12 hours. When used only at bedtime during the worst 2 to 3 days of a cold, it can make a world of difference. Everyone feels better after a good night's sleep. It is extremely effective and unblocks the nose in seconds without the systemic side effects of oral decongestants. However, it is tempting to overuse it since it works so well. When used properly, it is the best way I know to weather a cold.

Another suggestion is to try spraying only one nostril. That can be sufficient to allow your child to breathe comfortably. Spray the alternate nostril the next night. Apply a coat of Vaseline to the inside of the nostrils to prevent excessive drying and, as always, give plenty of fluids.

I've always heard that you can get "addicted" to nose sprays, so I never would use them myself much less give them to my daughter. Am I right?

I only wish parents felt that way about antibiotics! Most parents have never used Afrin themselves much less given it to their kids for fear of "rebound congestion" or dependence. This is not a problem with short-term, intermittent usage.

COUGH MEDICINES

Coughing is a protective reflex to clear the airways. Since most coughs are best left untreated, it's just as well that medications aren't too good at suppressing them. Although protective in the initial phases of an illness, a cough frequently lingers longer than it needs to. The reason for this is that coughing itself causes some "microtrauma" to the tissues. This irritation provokes further coughing and begins a vicious cycle. It is not uncommon for coughs to last for weeks after the initiating illness has resolved. In this case, medication may be appropriate, especially at bedtime when coughs are most bothersome.

Dextromethorphan is indicated by a "D" or "DM" found on most cough or cold medications. It is safe and widely available, but it must not work very well or the doctor's waiting room wouldn't be so crowded with coughing children (i.e., mom has already tried it).

Codeine is a much better cough suppressant, but it is a narcotic like morphine or heroin and can cause dependency. A lot of children get stomachaches from codeine and young children can stop breathing. Like Afrin, I use it with caution in older children during the worst two or three nights of a particularly bad cold and coughing. For obvious reasons, a prescription is required.

Benadryl (diphenhydramine) is a good cough suppressant in its own right, and its sedating and antiallergic effects add to its usefulness. The recommended dose on the label, however, is too low. Ask your doctor how much Benadryl is safe for your child. It is an all-around good choice for most lingering, nagging coughs.

EXPECTORANTS

Guaifenesin is the only expectorant found in cough and cold medicines such as Robitussin. The *Physicians' Desk Reference* states that guaifenesin is supposed to "enhance the output of lower respiratory tract fluid." To the best of my knowledge there is no medical evidence that it actually does this. In any case, the "lower respiratory tract" refers to the lungs, and I wouldn't depend on guaifenesen if I had pneumonia, bronchitis, or asthma. The lower respiratory tract isn't even involved when mucus from a cold or allergy is clogging the throat.

COMBINATION COLD FORMULAS

It is common knowledge that there is no cure for the common cold, but many people still seem to think that their doctor has a prescription that will make them feel better—something "stronger" than found in the drugstore. It's just not true. I get bad colds, too. The pharmacy shelves are packed with dozens of medications that attempt to relieve cold symptoms.

All these formulas contain various combinations and concentrations of the same basic ingredients: decongestants, antihistamines, cough suppressants, expectorants, and pain relievers. Including an expectorant to loosen secretions so thay can be coughed up in the same bottle with a cough suppressant or including an antihistamine to dry secretions in the same bottle with an expectorant to loosen them makes no sense. However, many formulas do exactly that.

If they don't work well, why are there so many of them?
Exactly. If some of them actually worked, there wouldn't be so many. Manufacturers keep reshuffling the same ingredients, change the name and flavor, and market it as a new product. When you're miserable with a cold and you see "new and improved," you go for it.

How come they are still on the market?
You keep buying them.

You really don't have anything stronger you can write me a prescription for?
No of course not. Do you think I just don't want you to have it? Cold formulas that require a prescription have codeine in them or have one of the newer antihistamines that have serious drug interactions and must be used with caution. If I think that one of these is warranted, I just prescribe the codeine or antihistamine by itself. You don't want all that other junk they put in them.

But what about codeine?

Codeine can make children feel better and not just when they have a cold either (Why do you think they call it dope?), but it's addictive and can cause stomachaches and respiratory depression. In older kids I do prescribe it for 2 to 3 days for coughs that just won't quit, hoping to interrupt the vicious cough cycle.

What about menthol, eucalyptus, and camphor?

Laboratory studies have shown that these substances do not increase airflow in the nose (i.e., relieve congestion). However, they can stimulate sensors in the nose that make you *think* you are breathing easier. Lozenges promote saliva production that can thin and wash down mucous secretions, but so can Life Savers. A chest rub has merits all its own. People do report feeling better and I guess that's what counts after all, isn't it?

Cold formulas seem to help my child. How do you explain that?

It may be that your child is allergic and you're giving her something containing an antihistamine. If it contains no decongestant, it may be making her sleepy and she's resting better—that always helps. Plain old Benadryl would do the same thing.

Read the labels. Buy a cold medicine she likes, is cheap, and doesn't have any extra medications in it that she doesn't need. I would especially avoid any with a decongestant. The last thing you need is a hyper, miserable kid with a cold.

Medications for Vomiting and Diarrhea

VOMITING

Vomiting is a protective mechanism to rid the body of noxious substances, usually viruses, bad food, poisons, or bacteria. It is a nonspecific symptom, and children can vomit even if the offensive agent is in their throats, lungs, kidneys, ears, blood, etc. The treatment for vomiting is to treat its underlying cause.

Vomiting usually lasts less than 24 hours, often less than 12 hours. Older children may vomit only once or twice. The best thing to do when your child vomits is to wait it out. It doesn't last that long and it may actually be helping him get over what ails him. If the vomiting lasts longer or gets progressively more frequent, the cause should be more carefully sought. Intractable vomiting can be a concern in and of itself as well as a symptom of more serious illness.

In some few cases it may be advisable to treat protracted vomiting. An antiemetic such as Phenergan (promethazine) can be given by intramuscular injection or as a suppository. I use this for small children who may be in imminent danger of dehydrating before an appropriate diagnosis is made and treatment of the primary illness instituted.

I have some leftover Phenergan suppositories in my refrigerator. If my son vomits, could I use one until I can get in touch with my doctor?

This is not a good idea for a couple of reasons. First of all, vomiting is a symptom of an underlying illness and not the illness itself. It would not be advisable to drug him (Phenergan is a good antiemetic but is also a major tranquilizer) because this could alter his mental status and make it difficult for the doctor to determine what is going on. Second, vomiting almost always subsides in 24 hours no matter what the cause, and most of the time a child will only vomit a couple of times anyway. The sedative effect of Phenergan can last all day.

What about Emetrol?

No parent has ever told me that Emetrol stopped their child's vomiting. If it did, it was probably because the vomiting was over anyway. It is supposed to be given in very small (teaspoonful) doses at 15-minute intervals. I think it is just something to do while waiting for the vomiting to run its course.

Then what can I do?

A better choice would be to offer a replacement fluid such as Pedialyte or Gatorade in the same small doses over 5- or 10-minute intervals to help prevent dehydration. The child may vomit that also, but if you keep trying, sooner or later he will keep it down and recovery is on the way.

DIARRHEA

Like vomiting, diarrhea is the body's attempt to get rid of an offensive agent. However, diarrhea is more specific than vomiting and usually signifies something is wrong with the gastrointestinal tract. As with vomiting, diarrhea is treated by treatment of the underlying cause.

Diarrhea frequently follows vomiting and can last many more days. So in addition to treating the primary illness, fluid replacement becomes more important. Several commercial fluid replacement drinks are made for young children (e.g., Pedialyte). Sports drinks (e.g., Gatorade or Powerade) and whatever foods they can tolerate are usually satisfactory for older kids.

Frequently the body's protective mechanisms overdo it. The gut continues to "wash out" the offensive agent long after it has disappeared. When diarrhea is still "out of control" several days into the illness and the cause is established and appropriate treatment (if needed) is begun, it is reasonable to try one or two doses of Imodium A-D (loperamide) in children older than 1 year. This "paralyzes" the gut temporarily, and most of the time slows things down considerably.

What about Kaopectate and other medications the pharmacist recommends for diarrhea?

Kaopectate, Donnagel, and Diasorb are supposed to adsorb offensive agents from the intestine to curb diarrhea. I have seen no evidence that they work very well.

What about Pepto-Bismol?

Since Pepto-Bismol is an aspirin-like compound, it may make you feel better for the same reasons aspirin does, but it is not recommended for use in children because of its theoretical link with Reye's syndrome. It is also an antimicrobial and may actually kill some of the germs that cause diarrhea. This takes time though and relief (if any) is delayed. I avoid its use in children because of its aspirin-like effects. It's worth a try for adult diarrhea.

Antibiotics

For decades, antibiotics were considered wonder drugs, but unfortunately the honeymoon is over. Anyone who's seen *Jurassic Park* knows that life will find a way. As fast as drug manufacturers develop new antibiotics, bacteria develop new methods of resistance.

How do the bacteria develop resistance to antibiotics?

Because bacteria grow quickly and exponentially, new genetic variants evolve by natural selection. If there were no antibiotic in the environment, a new variant wouldn't be anything special and would have to compete with its peers. In the presence of an antibiotic, however, its susceptible peers are eliminated and the resistant variant goes on to reproduce unchecked, giving rise to subsequent generations of resistant bacteria. Drug companies spend a lot of time and money to develop new drugs that bacteria can become resistant to in a few generations (days). It is not surprising that the microbes are winning the war against antimicrobials.

Isn't it just a matter of time until the problem of bacterial resistance to antibiotics is solved?

Microbes aren't likely to get dumber, but physicians and their patients can get wiser. The only way to slow the development of bacterial resistance is to stop selecting out resistant organisms by the casual use of antibiotics:

- Don't treat viral illnesses (upper respiratory infections, influenza, most sore throats and pneumonias, croup, and bronchiolitis) or allergic diseases (asthma and hay fever) with antibiotics.
- Don't try to kill every germ. It'll never happen. Use antibiotics with specificity for the infecting organism.
- Don't use antibiotics for any longer than absolutely necessary.
- Don't use preventive antibiotics. Think about it. It might work, but how would you know since your child might not have gotten sick anyway? If it doesn't work, by definition, you've created a resistant organism.

Is the situation really that bad?

Yes. In closed settings such as hospitals and in immunocompromised patients (newborns, elderly, and patients with AIDS or cancer) the problem of antibiotic resistance has already resulted in increased morbidity and mortality.

Could it happen to an otherwise healthy child?

Yes. *Any* antibiotic use can result in bacterial resistance.

What about taking the full 10-day course and finishing the medicine?

Except for more serious, but uncommon infections, this rule only applies to strep throat and even that may be changing. Almost everything else is negotiable. Ask your doctor.

You've convinced me, but how do I know if my son really needs an antibiotic?

Let your doctor know how you feel. A wait and see approach frequently pays off. You can always change your mind later. Ask for a painkiller instead. Your doctor will insist on antibiotics if your child really needs them.

My doctor says that my son needs an antibiotic. How do I know if he's prescribing the right one?

If a pediatrician decides to use an antibiotic, there are four basic classes to choose from:

- Penicillins, including amoxicillin and Augmentin
- Cephalosporins, including Ceclor, Cefzil, Cefobid, Ceftin, Vantin, Lorabid, and Cedax (the "cepha somethings")
- Erythromycins, including Pediazole, Ilosone, Biaxin, and Zithromax
- Sulfas, including Bactrim, Septra, and Pediazole

No one class is any "stronger" than another, and within classes no particular drug is necessarily any stronger than the others. It either kills the germ you're trying to kill or it doesn't. Each antibiotic has its own individual profile for coverage of specific germs and even drugs in the same class have some differences. Without a culture of the infected site and drug sensitivity testing, choosing the best antibiotic is just an educated guess.

Then why don't doctors just do a culture and choose the best antibiotic for the job?

Culturing infected tissue sites usually requires a needle puncture or other invasive procedure. A culture and sensitivity report from the lab takes at least 2 or 3 days and frequently longer. For these reasons, pediatricians usually have to make a decision without this information. However, although this approach has worked pretty well in the past, many hospitals and other settings now *require* physicians to do a culture and and get a sensitivity test before prescribing certain antibiotics.

Then how does the pediatrician decide?

They depend on data compiled in clinical studies and laboratory reports of infections occurring in the community. To date, the consensus is that amoxicillin is the best all-around first choice for common pediatric infections. No other single drug will work the first time more often than amoxicillin.

Amoxicillin never works for my son. Why can't we just go to the stronger stuff?

It is likely that your son has received amoxicillin in the past for viral rather than bacterial illnesses. There is still no other single drug that will work the first time more often than amoxicillin. There are some pockets (mostly in big cities) where amoxicillin is not considered the first choice for common pediatric infections. However, if this is the case, your pediatrician would be using the alternate recommended drug for that location for all his patients and not just your son.

If amoxicillin has failed as the first-line drug, there is no agreement on the best second choice. As far as picking the right drug for the germ, it's still just a guess. However, several factors are considered in choosing the next drug.

Taste
Cost
Dosing and length of therapy
Side effects
Drug allergies
Interactions with other medications
Interactions with food
Previous antibiotic usage
Known drug resistance patterns in the community

These factors vary and there is no universal second choice. Here are a few things it's good to know about the second-line antibiotics:

- All antibiotics can cause diarrhea, but Augmentin seems to do so more often than the others. Try to use the lowest effective dose and to space the doses as much as possible.
- All antibiotics can cause allergic skin reactions, but Ceclor does so more often than the others. This can happen even if it didn't with previous courses of the medication. It can also happen weeks after the medication is discontinued. As the newer "cepha somethings" are prescribed more frequently, there will probably be more reported cases of other drugs in this class causing allergic reactions.
- All antibiotics can upset the stomach, but the erythromycins are more likely to do so. Erythromycins cannot be taken concurrently with some of the newer antihistamines such as Seldane.
- People who have a true drug allergy to penicillin are also more likely to have an allergy to other antibiotics, particularly the cephalosporins. Multiple drug allergies are common.
- Sulfa drugs are some of the oldest antibiotics but aren't used much anymore. For this reason, they can work well. I use them often when they are indicated. They don't work for strep throat.
- All antibiotics can contribute to secondary yeast infections, especially diaper rash in babies.
- Cephalosporins taste the best, but a couple of these drugs have to be taken on an empty stomach. Lorabid is delicious, but it has to be taken twice a day either an hour before or 2 hours after eating. Try that on your child for 10 days!
- All the newer antibiotics are outrageously expensive.

What is the difference between drug side effects and drug allergies?

There is a big difference between drug side effects and drug allergic reactions. All drugs have the potential to cause side effects in any person; therefore it is the drug's "fault." Most side effects are just a nuisance, but some few can be life threatening. (If a drug frequently causes serious side effects, it wouldn't be on the market except in unusual circumstances.) If a patient experiences side effects, it is a judgment call whether to stop the medication or not. The drug can be used again in the future and the side effects may or may not recur.

On the other hand, allergic reactions (which can range from mild itching on one occasion to shock and death on another even in the same individual) are the result of a patient's immune system perceiving the antibiotic as a foreign invader; it is the patient's "fault." The antibiotic must be discontinued immediately and its use avoided in the future.

My son has a history of ear infections. My doctor asks *me* which antibiotic I want to give him. How should I know? He's the doctor!

Since it's a matter of trial and error, a parent can be very helpful in evaluating the various pros and cons of the second-line antibiotics. Mom knows which ones have worked well or caused problems in the past. Her input is valuable to the pediatrician in choosing the next drug. Fortunately, as time goes by, the child frequently gets well all by himself despite what we do.

What about a "shot"?

There are only two commonly used "shots" in pediatric medicine. One is Bicillin (a long-acting penicillin), which is used to treat strep throat in vomiting kids who can't keep oral penicillin down. Injections hurt and contrary to popular belief do not work any faster or better. (Actually the antibiotic gets into the bloodstream a few minutes later, but so what?) The advantage is that it is a "one shot deal" and can prevent reinfection for up to 3 weeks. Bicillin is still a useful option in treating strep throat.

The other newer shot is ceftriaxone (Rocephin). It is a broad-spectrum antibiotic (the kind you're supposed to avoid) and is generally used to quickly get medicine into children who you think might have a significant illness but the cause hasn't been determined yet. It is only effective for 24 hours, but this buys time until culture results are available. It can also be used for a day or two in children who are vomiting. Once oral medication can be tolerated and culture results are known, more specific antibiotic therapy can be instituted.

Can my son develop resistance to the antibiotics?

No, your son won't, but his germs will. It may be the same thing to you, but it's not to me. This will happen with any antibiotic, not just amoxicillin.

Will all this antibiotic usage "weaken his system"?

I think I know what you mean. No, his body doesn't get lazy and let the antibiotics do all the work for him. However, all antibiotics have side effects and these can add up and eventually take a toll on him but not the germs, unfortunately.

Key Points

- Antibiotics are not usually the answer to most pediatric problems and should be avoided except when absolutely necessary.
- It is reasonable to adopt a wait and see attitude. You can always change your mind later.
- If your doctor recommends amoxicillin, don't think that he is trivializing your child's complaint.
- Your child probably won't need to take a full 10-day course except for a few uncommon illnesses. Try to get by with less. Ask your doctor.
- Most antibiotics share the same kinds of side effects. Don't blame a particular one.
- Antibiotics not only affect your child but the entire community.

Antiviral Agents

Unlike antibiotics, the more recent discovery of antiviral agents has produced disappointing results. Viruses are so simple they depend on and cannot survive without a human host. There are limited ways of attacking the virus without also attacking the human. Bacteria are more complex organisms and there are more opportunities to attack them. At best, antiviral agents slow a virus down a little more than they slow the patient down. It is still up to the patient to get rid of the virus.

There are no wonder drugs in the antiviral world. They may lessen the impact of an infection or speed recovery by a day or so, but it is never dramatic. They are used in children with underlying conditions or those who are so sick that they require hospitalization. They have been very helpful in treating herpesvirus infections of the eyes that have the potential to cause significant loss of vision or blindness.

In otherwise healthy children there is little use for routine antiviral therapy. Occasionally it is used for chickenpox and shingles, other herpesvirus infections, and influenza. Several drugs are fairly good at *preventing* a specific viral illness such as influenza or genital herpes.

ACYCLOVIR FOR CHICKENPOX AND SHINGLES

Chickenpox is caused by the varicella-zoster virus, a member of the ubiquitous herpes family. Everyone knows about chickenpox, but there's a lot of confusion about shingles. Shingles, a painful eruption of blisters, occurs when the original chickenpox virus re-emerges from its hiding place in the nervous system—perhaps years later. Basically you "catch it" from yourself. Those with active lesions can spread it to anyone who hasn't already had chickenpox. Both chickenpox and shingles run their course in otherwise healthy children.

I've heard that there's a cure for chickenpox now. Some doctors prescribe this medicine over the phone and some say it doesn't work and won't prescribe it at all. Which is true?

In 1992 the Federal Drug Administration approved oral acyclovir for treating varicella infections in otherwise healthy kids. It is considered safe and will "impact favorably" on the course of the illness when given in the first 24 hours of the onset of the rash. It is expensive and must be given every 6 hours for 5 days. The Committee on Infectious Diseases of the American Academy of Pediatrics does *not* recommend the routine use of oral acyclovir for uncomplicated varicella. The committee believes that a "marginal" improvement in the course of the disease does not justify the high cost of acyclovir and that getting it to 4 million children a year in the first 24 hours of the onset of the rash is not feasible.

It's approved for routine use but not recommended. What, then, does a parent do?

Since 1992 it has been left to the pediatrician to decide with due consideration of the parent's wishes. Now that the chickenpox vaccine (Varivax) has been approved and is in general use, giving acyclovir for this condition may no longer be an issue. In the meantime I prescribe acyclovir in the first 24 hours if the parent requests it and recommend it for teenagers and others with special needs.

Does using acyclovir increase or decrease the chance of getting chicken-pox or shingles again?

There is no indication that this is so. By the time the rash of chickenpox or shingles appears, the virus has been replicating in the body for several days and the immune system has already had a chance to "kick in." However, with or without acyclovir, some patients do have a recurrence.

What did you do for your own children?

I was anticipating the breakout of the rash and was able to start acyclovir in the first few hours. I think that it made a difference in how they actually felt. If you can't start the medication right away, it's probably not worth it. Had the vaccine been available, I would have used it.

What about side effects?

They are minor, and no single side effect is especially noteworthy.

ACYCLOVIR FOR OTHER HERPESVIRUS INFECTIONS, INCLUDING MONONUCLEOSIS

Other viruses in the herpes family behave much like chickenpox. They remain dormant in the nervous system and can re-emerge at any time. This is the case with ulcers on the lips (cold sores or fever blisters) or genitals of children infected with herpesvirus types 1 and 2, respectively. Acyclovir can be applied topically to the ulcers and it may speed healing, but it is not as effective as taking pills every 6 hours. Oral acyclovir can be used in some instances depending on the severity and frequency of "outbreaks," but it is usually not worth it. An exception would be using long-term prophylactic acyclovir in teenagers with frequent, recurrent genital herpes who are sexually active.

In young children, usually under 2 years of age, several other very common infections are caused by herpesviruses (e.g., roseola and gingivostomatitis). So far acyclovir has not been effective in treating these benign, but anxiety-producing illnesses. They still "just have to run their course."

I've seen an ad on TV for a new drug to treat genital herpes. What's that all about?

Valtrex (valacyclovir) is a drug similar to acyclovir that can be taken less often (every 12 hours) instead of every 4 to 6 hours. It can make prophylactic therapy of genital herpes simpler in those patients who elect to do so.

What about acyclovir for Epstein-Barr virus, mononucleosis, and chronic fatigue syndrome?

Infectious mononucleosis is caused by the Epstein-Barr virus, which belongs to the herpes family. To date, studies of acyclovir for the treatment of mononucleosis are inconclusive. It may be worth a try if the child is really sick. The role of Ebstein-Barr virus (if any) in chronic fatigue syndrome is still so uncertain that I wouldn't recommend acyclovir.

FLUMADINE FOR INFLUENZA

There are many influenza viruses, but they can be divided into two basic types, influenza A and influenza B. Each year several types run rampant around the globe. Healthy people do okay, but weak ones can die. Yearly vaccination is the best way to avoid influenza.

I hear some people say there's treatment for flu and some say there isn't. Who's right?

Both and neither. Influenza A can be treated but not influenza B. If your child gets influenza A, Flumadine (rimantidine) can be helpful if started in the first 24 hours of the illness, but like all antivirals, it is no wonder drug. It is not curative, but it may lessen the symptoms and shorten the duration of the illness.

Technically speaking, Flumadine is only approved for *prevention* and not treatment of influenza A infection. Influenza virus circulates at about the same time as other common respiratory viruses, and in the early days of a febrile illness in a young child it is hard to differentiate them. Even if you "test" for influenza on the very first day, the lab results may not get back for 24 hours. In addition, most moms don't rush their child to the doctor's office in the first hours that he feels ill. By the time you can get the medicine to a child, it is often too late to make a difference.

Who should receive preventive Flumadine therapy?

The same ones who should have been vaccinated. If for some reason, a high-risk child was not vaccinated, Flumadine can be used until the vaccination is given and has had time to become effective (usually 2 to 4 weeks). Again, Flumadine will not prevent influenza B.

Can anyone who chooses be vaccinated for influenza or do you have to be in some high-risk category?

Almost anyone can be vaccinated. It makes more sense to do this than use Flumadine. The vaccine is more effective and will cover more of the circulating strains since it also covers influenza B. I would rather the entire family be vaccinated once a year than have them all use Flumadine twice a day for weeks and then succumb to influenza B. If you decide to get a vaccination after influenza season is well under way, it makes sense to use Flumadine for a couple of weeks until the vaccine can take effect.

My daughter woke up sick this morning and I just know it's flu since her brother had it last week. Can you give her something?

She should have been vaccinated as soon as her brother was diagnosed and, if he had influenza A (based on community health reports), placed on Flumadine for prevention at that time. If he had influenza B, there is nothing that can be done now. Since you probably don't know if it's A or B, then it is worth trying Flumadine since you are "catching it" early.

How do you know if it is influenza A or B?

Without tests you can't know, and most labs report only "influenza" and do not specify type A or B. However, some labs and most health departments do surveillance testing and keep physicians updated on what strains are going around.

My child is sick with the flu even though he was vaccinated. Now what can I do?

Most likely it's not influenza at all but rather a flu-like illness. If it is a confirmed case of influenza, it could be from late vaccination or vaccine failure. Like all vaccines, influenza vaccine is about 70% to 90% effective, and it takes 2 to 4 weeks to "kick in." Rarely (once or twice in the last couple of decades) the experts guessed wrong and the vaccine did not cover the strains that circulated that year. If type A is circulating, Flumadine may be worth a try. If it is type B, he's going to be sick but not as sick as if he hadn't been vaccinated.

Antifungal Drugs

Antifungals are now readily available in over-the-counter creams, ointments, and powders for skin infections such as yeast diaper rashes, athlete's foot, and ringworm. They are all effective and do not have significant side effects. If your child's rash does not respond, it's probably not due to a fungus and you should consult your doctor.

Aren't prescription creams stronger?

The over-the-counter products work so well that it is usually not worth a trip to the doctor for a prescription for the newest antifungal drugs. If the other creams fail, there's a good chance that the problem is not caused by a fungus and they won't work either.

My son frequently gets athlete's foot from the showers at school and the over-the-counter creams aren't working anymore. Would a prescription cream work better?

Since your son and his friends have probably used the over-the-counter creams frequently in the past, the fungus may have developed some resistance. Prescription medications may be more effective.

My doctor says my newborn has thrush. How did she get that and what can I do about it?

Thrush is a yeast (type of fungus) infection found in the mouth of newborns that is acquired from their mothers when they pass through the birth canal. Nystatin oral suspension is the mainstay of treatment along with good hygienic practices. You need a prescription. Gentian violet, a purple dye available without prescription, works but is very messy. Both nystatin and gentian violet are "painted on" the cheeks, gums, tongue, and lips and are not meant to be swallowed. But if your baby swallows some by accident, it won't hurt her. A new prescription medication called Diflucan (fluconazole) works much better. It is taken orally and acts systemically so there is a potential for side effects. If nystatin or gentian violet fail after a couple of weeks, Diflucan is worth a try.

My daughter has ringworm on her scalp. Will the over-the-counter antifungal creams treat it?

No. "Deep" fungal infections of the scalp, nails, and skin require long-term oral antifungal therapy. Topical (even prescription) medication is not effective. Griseofulvin is still the drug of choice, but it can have serious side effects and its use must be monitored carefully. Oral ketoconazole and others may soon replace it, but they also have some serious drawbacks and must be used cautiously.

Steroids

Steroids are a large class of drugs that have common molecular similarities but very different effects on the body. They can be classified roughly according to the organ systems they affect the most. For instance, anabolic steroids such as testosterone can build muscles but have little anti-inflammatory effects. Glucocorticosteroids such as hydrocortisone are good anti-inflammatory drugs but won't build muscle.

This gets even more confusing when the various concentrations and strengths are taken into account. Steroids have limited and well-defined uses in pediatric medicine, namely, to treat allergic diseases (such as asthma, hay fever, or eczema), allergic reactions (such as poison ivy, hives, or reactions to penicillin), and occasionally viral infectious diseases (croup or mononucleosis).

To make things simple, I will use the word "steroid" to represent glucocorticosteroids that are used for their anti-inflammatory properties (e.g., hydrocortisone, prednisone, and dexamethasone). Steroids can be given as intravenous or intramuscular injections, taken orally in tablet or liquid form, or applied directly to the skin as a cream or ointment. They can also be inhaled into the lungs or nose or used as eyedrops.

Dosing is inexact at best and can better be thought of as small, medium, or large. There are dozens of steroids with many similar properties that can be used interchangeably but require dosing adjustments. For example, prednisone and dexamethasone do the same things, but five times more prednisone than dexamethasone is needed to accomplish the same task. To confuse things even more, 1% hydrocortisone cream is many hundred times *weaker* than let's say 0.05% of a fluorinated steroid cream. Get it? Most people (and even physicians) don't, so they use charts that categorize the various steroids into weak, stronger, and strongest. All steroids in the same category have equivalent effects and can be used interchangeably, especially since dosing isn't a precise science.

Most physicians become familiar with a couple of the least expensive steroids in each category and use them over and over. Many hospitals, insurance companies, and health plans only approve of a limited formulary of drugs in each category. Generally the generic ones are cheaper, and there's no good reason to buy the expensive brand name products. Because there are so many names, concentrations, forms, strengths, and prices, many patients receive a different one every time they see a doctor for the exact same problem. It's no wonder patients are confused.

Every time I take my son to the doctor for eczema I get different sample tubes of medicine. Which one is really the best?

The doctor is doing you a favor by giving you medication for free and also saving you a trip to the drugstore. Most of the samples left by the drug representatives are of medium potency, and there is so little difference among them that it won't make a difference to your child, especially since you probably are not very precise in the amount you use each time. The low-potency steroids are available without a prescription and aren't marketed to physicians. There are few if any indications for using the highest potency steroids in children, and pediatricians usually do not get sample tubes of these.

Why are the tubes so small?

Because they are samples, but it's a good thing since steroids are recommended to be used sparingly and only for short periods of time. They work very well, but if used indiscriminately, there is the risk of side effects or complications.

Why are there so many different steroids and why do they have so many side effects?

Steroids are highly potent drugs that can affect almost every cell of the body. The reason there are so many is that drug companies keep trying to custom design steroids to affect some specific cells and leave the rest alone. For example, it would be great if inflammation in the lungs of asthmatics could be effectively treated without signaling the liver to raise the blood sugar level. So far there has not been much success, and that is why the list of side effects and potential complications from steroid use is so long.

Is it safe to use steroids in children?

Fortunately, the side effects of steroids in children are not as worrisome as they are in adults, who tend to have diseases in addition to that which requires steroid therapy—heart disease, high blood pressure, glaucoma, depression, and diabetes to name a few. The only side effect that is a major concern in healthy children is the potential of steroids to suppress the body's infection-fighting abilities (immunosuppression). This is the greatest concern in asthmatic children who require frequent, intermittent, or long-term steroid use.

My son is asthmatic and occasionally has to take oral prednisone. Does this make him more susceptible to colds and other infectious illnesses?

Theoretically, steroids can weaken the body's defenses against all infections, but only infections caused by members of the herpesvirus family (including chickenpox) and influenza pose any serious problem on a regular basis. Even though there are now vaccines for chickenpox and influenza, pediatricians are still careful about prescribing steroids if there is any possibility of infection. Your son, however, is at much greater risk from his asthma than from steroid-induced immunosuppression.

Then why would a steroid be used for an infectious illness such as croup or mononucleosis?

Surprisingly, steroids are occasionally recommended for illnesses caused by infections. This is true for the viral illnesses croup and mononucleosis. In an infant with croup the airway can swell so much that breathing is severely restricted. Steroids can reduce the swelling (again a trade-off between decreasing inflammation at the cost of immunosuppression). In some cases of mononucleosis it is not the virus itself that makes the person feel so bad (especially after the first week or so) but the body's "overreacting" to it. Steroids can quell the inflammatory response. In general, as far as infectious disease is concerned, as long as the body's defenses are well under way in their fight against the infection, steroids probably won't hurt and may help the patient feel better sooner.

• • •

If your doctor puts your child on steroids, here are a few things you should know:

Steroid creams and ointments for dermatitis or eczema should be used sparingly for only short periods of time. A medium potency should be used on the body and if possible a low potency on the face, although occasionally a medium potency may be required. Applying a tight diaper over the cream or ointment will significantly increase the penetration into the skin and usually should be avoided. Ointments and gels are better than creams for penetrating thick, leathery skin. There is little risk of any side effects with these kinds of steroids. Some flare-up is to be expected after stopping treatment. To prevent a vicious cycle, try to wait it out. Incidentally, 1% hydrocortisone cream (Cortaid) is great for first aid for insect or spider bites.

Steroid nasal sprays for allergic rhinitis can often control a child's seasonal allergies. Use one spray in each nostril once or twice a day during the allergic periods. The sprays come in different cannisters, and some are more difficult to handle than others. Some preparations also cause more burning and sneezing. Trying the doctor's samples before you buy can help in making the best choice. Again, there is little risk and frequently there is significant relief when these steroid sprays are used as directed.

Steroid eyedrops are used like steroid nasal sprays and some burn more than others. They must be used with caution, however, since your child may be at significant risk if she has a viral infection (specifically herpesvirus infection) of the eyes instead of or in addition to allergic conjunctivitis. It is difficult to tell the difference and most pediatricians won't prescribe steroid eyedrops for this reason. They leave it to an ophthalmologist after a careful eye examination.

Inhaled steroid drugs for the treatment of asthma are also used once or twice a day just like steroid nasal sprays. They are very effective and the risk of immunosuppression is small. Inhaled steroids are reserved for those kids whose asthma is difficult to control by other means since the risk of a severe life-threatening asthma attack outweighs the risk of infection. Also, controlling asthma in itself decreases the risk of secondary infection. Such children should be vaccinated for chickenpox and influenza.

Short courses (4 to 7 days) of oral steroids are used to treat poison ivy, poison oak, hives, or any other allergic skin manifestation that is persistent. Many of these conditions subside over time without treatment, and the risks and benefits in a particular patient must be weighed carefully. Applying topical steroids to the skin lesions themselves will *not* alter the course of a systemic allergic reaction. Occasional use of steroids for skin conditions carries little risk unless the child has not yet had chickenpox (and has not been vaccinated) or during influenza season. Fortunately, influenza and poison ivy seasons do not usually overlap.

Oral steroids are prescribed in "tapering doses." A larger 24-hour dose is taken for the first couple of days and decreased gradually every day or two. There are no precise guidelines for dosing and physicians differ in the regimen they prefer. The total daily dose can be divided into two or three smaller doses or taken all at once with food in the morning (even better). I divide the dose if the patient doesn't like taking several pills or ounces of medication at once. Medically, it's probably better to take a single large dose, but that's splitting hairs.

When a steroid is used for croup, it is usually given in a single injection. Oral steroids will work just as well, but these children have a lot of respiratory distress (that's why they are getting the shot in the first place), and an injection is the easiest and fastest way to give a lot of medication. Also, children may resist drinking large volumes of medication or may vomit it up.

Steroids for infectious mononucleosis remain controversial. I prescribe them for teenagers who seem to be sicker than most. They seem to make a difference sometimes, but not frequently.

It's important to know that the effects of steroids can last several months after taking the last dose. Health care personnel attending to your child need to be informed of current and previous steroid use. If your child develops any other medical problems while taking steroids, call your doctor.

4

You and Your Newborn

I often tell new mothers in my office, "If you study the baby as carefully as the baby *books*, you wouldn't need them." Motherhood is learned from babies not from books.

A new mother simply needs to love her baby and trust her natural maternal instincts. It is easy for her to love her baby, but trusting her maternal instincts in today's culture is a lot more difficult. The natural instincts of motherhood have been bombarded by a blitz of information, misinformation, and noninformation on the "right" way to raise a baby. A mom is usually bewildered by what she *feels* is the right thing to do and what she has been *told* is the right thing to do.

This chapter is certainly not meant to tell you everything about taking care of your baby. In fact, just the opposite. I'd rather you spend the time with the baby and just do what feels right. For those who must have a more definitive roadmap, go ahead and visit the child care section of your local bookstore. If *you* don't have any ideas on how to raise your baby, the ones you find in the many books available are just as good as any. If you think you can go it alone, this chapter is meant to offer you some reassurance. I think you will get the idea in just a few pages. Some legitimate medical questions will be addressed that keep coming up repeatedly in the office. Obviously the many baby books have failed to cover some basic concerns.

Feeding

Although newborn infants expect to be breast-fed on demand, they will thrive on breast milk, formula, or a combination of the two. In time you and your baby will arrive at an arrangement that works well for both of you and don't let anyone tell you differently. If it seems to be a struggle at first, just remind yourself that she is programmed to be breast-fed on demand and anything else is a stretch for her. Take it a day at a time and be flexible until you arrive at a satisfactory schedule.

I know that breast is best, but I have to give my baby formula. Which is the closest to breast milk?

A newborn can grow well on any of the standard baby formulas containing iron. Special formulas, vitamins, or fluoride are not needed unless certain medical conditions indicate their use.

Iron makes me constipated and gaseous. Why would I give it to my baby?

Iron is an important component of red blood cells and muscle cells and is not a special additive as the label may suggest. Most new mothers have taken or may still be taking iron prescribed by their OB/GYN during their pregnancy. Extra iron is needed to meet the demands of the pregnancy and the rapid growth of the baby. These big pills are taken once or twice a day and they make most gaseous, constipated pregnant women even more so. Baby formula contains only the amount of iron the baby needs and is meted out in small doses when the baby feeds.

What about fluoride?

Fluoride, occurring naturally to varying degrees in water, is usually added to most municipal water supplies. There is no way of knowing how much fluoride is present in food or drinks commercially prepared with water (it is not found on the label). Mom delivers the fluoride she has consumed to her breast-fed infant. Too much fluoride stains the teeth (fluorosis). When breast-fed babies were routinely given fluoride, there was a dramatic increase in fluorosis. Fluoride supplements are no longer recommended.

How long do I have to boil the water and sterilize the bottles and nipples?

You don't have to do this at all if your tap water is from an approved community water supply and not a private well. Your baby is not sterile and neither are you. Good handwashing and dishwashing practices are good enough for newborns.

What about using bottled water?

If you prefer to use bottled water for whatever reason, fine. Just remember that an approved community water supply may be more carefully monitored than a bottled water supply (they are not regulated). I've seen Gerber baby water on the supermarket shelves. Really!

My doctor told me to change to soy formula when my baby gets diarrhea. It doesn't seem to help. Is it really necessary?

No. There are some legitimate medical reasons to change formulas, but simple, occasional diarrhea isn't one of them. Babies are not meant to be fed a varied diet, and it is unwise to casually switch formulas every time he fusses, cries, screams, spits, vomits, "poops" too much or too little, cramps or passes gas, or stays up too late, in other words "acts like a baby."

I know that soy comes from soybeans and milk from cows. Does this make any difference to my baby?

Not really. Humans are probably more cow-like than bean-like, but it is amazing how similar plants and animals really are. All living organisms use the same 20 amino acids to make the proteins they need. Your baby can get these "building blocks" from either source. Both formulas contain the same amount of iron and are equally nutritious. Although allergic reactions are uncommon, infants can be allergic to cow protein, soy protein, or both. The sugar in cow's milk (lactose) is the same as that in breast milk; however, the "predigested" sugar in soy formula may be easier on an infant after a *prolonged* bout of diarrhea. If you switch from cow's milk to soy for that reason, remember that you are introducing a new protein to your child's "recovering" gastrointestinal tract. It may not be such a good idea, but many pediatricians do it automatically when an infant gets diarrhea. Remember that human breast milk is always preferred when practical.

How much breast milk or formula is enough?

Don't watch the clock; watch the baby and he will let you know. Don't be compelled to finish off the bottle. If he pulls away and turns his head, he's had enough. Remember that a baby will suck on anything placed in his mouth. It's a reflex and doesn't necessarily mean that he is hungry.

When should I start solid foods?

Most babies are ready for solid foods by 6 months of age. Although you can coax a younger baby to eat solids before then, it is more of a struggle and not usually necessary as long as she is growing. Babies do not even lose their protective tongue-thrust reflex until about 4 months of age, which accounts for the constant scooping back into the mouth of food deliberately spit out. (Maybe she's trying to tell you something.)

Won't solid foods help her sleep through the night?

No. Studies have shown over and over again that starting solid food will not increase the chance of your baby sleeping through the night.

I know I'm supposed to start with rice cereal, but what after that?

It doesn't really matter how you introduce solids. (Most of the rest of the world does not have the luxury of color-coded baby food jars lining the grocery store shelves). Just go slowly to see if your baby reacts to a new food. There's no hurry. It is okay to skip the jars altogether. There are enough iron-fortified cereals and mashable foods to keep a formula or breast-fed baby growing well until he can gum or chew table foods.

I can't get my baby to eat meat! What do you recommend?

If babies were meant to eat meat, they would have teeth. Wait until he can chew well. He gets all the protein and iron he needs from his milk and cereal.

Which foods are most likely to cause problems?

Most kids are not allergic to any food, but when they are the most common offenders are milk, berries, nuts, eggs, wheat, soybeans, and seafood. When introducing these for the first time, don't try any other new food for a few days so you can see if your child has a problem with these foods.

What about honey?

Honey is a definite no-no before the age of 12 months because of the risk of infant botulism. Older children can handle the *Clostridium* spores, but young ones can't.

What about sugar?

The body converts dietary sugar into glucose, the only form of sugar it can use for energy. Studies have shown many times over that sugar does not affect the behavior of children. Moderation is advised for all things, including sugar.

What about fruit juices?

Fruit juices are meant to be consumed with the fruit. You'd probably have to eat about 50 apples to get the equivalent of an 8-ounce bottle of apple juice. No wonder it gives kids diarrhea. If your child can tolerate it, okay, but don't be surprised if he can't. I use the 10% fruit juice drinks, especially the ones with added calcium and vitamin C. They contain mostly water with juice added to equal that found in a piece of fruit plus some other goodies. Apple juice (even 8 ounces) doesn't contain any appreciable vitamin C.

When can I stop using infant formula?

By the age of 12 months most children consume enough calories from table foods to permit them to be taken off calorie-rich infant formula. A breast-fed baby will adjust his own intake accordingly (mom's milk adjusts too). This is a good time to switch from formula to whole milk.

Do I have to change to whole milk gradually?

There is no dietary reason for this, but it may take some time for your baby to adjust to the taste. In kids who seem to be having trouble making the switch, try heating the milk or cooling it down. Some children never adjust because they just don't like milk. That's okay, too. Just make sure your baby gets other calcium-rich foods such as cheese, yogurt, and calcium-enriched juices.

When should I stop giving a bottle?

If you haven't already done so, start offering a cup when you switch to whole milk, but there's no reason to be rigid. As your child grows, the bottle will not deliver enough volume fast enough through the nipple to satisfy her. (Just don't make the holes bigger!) Puppies and kitties wean themselves. Always have a cup available, and your child will prefer that by the time she is 2 years or so. Your child usually prefers drinking out of *your* cup long before then.

What's the easiest way to wean my baby from the breast?

Weaning from the breast is more complex only because mother/infant pairs establish so many patterns of breast-feeding. Everyone starts the weaning process from a different place. Establish some goals and go for it. Baby is a lot tougher now, and it's okay to expect him to conform to your schedule. If you've managed to avoid bottles for the first 6 months or so, you can probably get by without ever having to introduce the bottle (he'd probably hate it anyway).

I'm sure I did it all wrong! Now what do I do?

No matter what feeding practices you established in the beginning, you can always expect some difficult transition periods. Don't blame yourself for not being tougher early on. You do the best you can under the circumstances. No one gets through it unscathed, and anyone who tells you differently is a liar!

Sleeping

Infants should be put to sleep on their backs, not propped on their sides with pillows or other soft bedding. Since the "back to sleep" campaign was begun, deaths from sudden infant death syndrome (SIDS) are down almost 30%.

At the 2-week checkup I typically hear moms say, "My baby's got her days and nights mixed up." I no longer hear this comment when the child is 2 months old. Obviously somewhere between 2 weeks and 2 months baby's sleep patterns get straightened out. Remember, newborns have spent the last 9 months in the dark and it will take some time to adjust to extrauterine light/dark cycles. Mammalian brains are highly sensitive to daily light/dark cycles and seasonal patterns. You may want to think twice about leaving the lights on at all hours.

Is it okay to let my baby sleep in my bed?

Sure. It helps to have the baby close by at night. Most people in the world (and the entire animal kingdom) don't have the luxury of separate bedrooms for their children. Bed sharing or room sharing is perfectly natural. Move the baby out when the advantages no longer outweigh the disadvantages. Expect the first few nights to be rough, but the early closeness and convenience were worth it.

Will I roll over on him?

I have never heard of this actually happening. (Does anyone ever sleep that soundly with a newborn in the bed?) You are a better judge of your sleeping habits.

When are babies supposed to sleep through the night?

Sleeping through the night is a developmental milestone like rolling over or walking. The range is from birth to about 2 years. You can't make it happen before it's time. You can delay it, however, by responding to baby's every stirring during the night. (Turn down the monitor!)

When can I stop feeding him during the night?

By 2 months of age or about 12 pounds babies are capable of going 6 to 8 hours without eating. It is reasonable to try to eliminate the nighttime feedings, but you can't make him sleep.

My baby is 3 months old and weighs 15 pounds. He's still waking up several times during the night and he's obviously hungry because he devours 8 ounces of milk. How can I stop feeding him if he is hungry?

If you feed your baby every time he arouses at night you are rewarding him for waking up. He thinks he is pleasing you. It's really okay to stop those nighttime feedings even if he screams bloody murder. Some babies catch on faster than others, but be patient. Soon he will eat more during the day and won't feel hungry during the night. Transition periods are always a little rough, so wait until you can handle this one. Remember that eliminating breast-feeding during the night may ultimately lead to earlier weaning. That's okay; it's just a choice you have to make.

I enjoy those peaceful, quiet 2 A.M. feedings. Am I wrong to continue them?

No, of course not. Many mothers actually do enjoy the quiet one-on-one 2 A.M. feedings. Keep it up if you like, but you may end up with an 18-month-old who still wants mommy and a bottle or breast at 2 A.M. even if he's not hungry (after all, *he* can take a nap tomorrow). It may be worth it to you to hang on to those precious moments. If you'd rather your baby sleep through the night, stop feeding him as soon as possible and make nighttime encounters brief and to the point.

How often should my baby nap?

Napping is extremely variable. It's reasonable to put the baby down a couple of times a day so you can have a life, but you can't make him sleep. A lot of babies don't need to nap much. They drive their mothers crazy and then go on to be very accomplished adults.

Does it help to keep him up as long as possible and then lay him down for a long nap?

This is rarely successful. Many moms try to "wear their babies out" with stimulating activities, but it's more likely that the mom will succumb first. Everything is stimulating and new to an infant so don't overdo "baby activities." Monotony and boredom are better precursors to sleep than sensory overload.

Hygiene
BATHING

How often should I bathe my baby?

Your baby doesn't have much opportunity to get dirty. After all, some-one is always wiping her mouth, hands, and bottom. Since the natural oils in her skin protect her from irritants in the environment, it's preferable to go several days or more between baths. She'll need a shampoo by then. Soap only the obviously dirty parts (use Dove soap), rinse her off, and get her out. Don't scrub off nature's protective coat. That includes the wax in her ears.

My newborn has very sensitive skin and gets a lot of rashes. What should I do?

It is best to leave your baby's skin alone. Babies can get lots of minor rashes as their skin adjusts to life outside the watery womb. Most babies will peel and get scaly skin in the first weeks after birth, and lotions will not prevent this. Overbathing and applying commercial products can cause some of the skin problems in infants.

DIAPERS

Are disposable or cloth diapers best?

Environmentally, it's a toss-up between cloth and disposable diapers. But you can't beat disposables for comfort, convenience, and hygiene. Dis-posable diapers are so good today that many older babies can get along fine with as few as three or so a day compared with 8 to 10 cloth diapers.

Elimination

Mothers suffer unnecessary anxiety about baby's stools. Unless the baby is sick or clearly uncomfortable or in pain, most stool patterns are acceptable.

My baby's bowel movements seem to cause him a lot of discomfort. Is something wrong?

Most babies grunt and groan, pull up their legs, strain, and turn red in the face when they have a bowel movement. (You probably would too if you tried to do it flat on your back.)

How often should he have a bowel movement?

Some breast-fed babies may have 8 to 10 bowel movements a day. Some are comfortable with none for a couple of weeks. Bottle babies are more "regular," but there is still a lot variability. Most *average* about one or two a day.

What color should the stools be?

Any color's okay except red (blood), black (tarry), or white (oatmeal).

My baby has a lot of gas. What can I do?

Nothing really. Some medications are available that claim to alleviate gas temporarily, but swallowing air while feeding and crying is an ongoing process. It's a losing battle.

When should I worry?

If there is a persistent, significant *change* in bowel habits or if there are other symptoms, call the doctor.

My baby's stools are infrequent and are always hard, round pellets. Is this okay?

A pattern of persistent hard stools that are passed infrequently is considered constipation. There are several causes, some of which can indicate a more serious problem and should be investigated by your doctor.

Common Problems in Newborns

"Never trust a neonate." This is one of the first things pediatric residents are taught. Infants under the age of 2 months do not always show traditional signs of illness and serious illness can go undetected. There is a long list of things that can go wrong. If you notice any change in your newborn's behavior that concerns you, call your doctor. It is likely your doctor will want to see him. Pediatricians frequently admit newborns to the hospital just to check them out. Most will not have a serious problem, but we don't want to miss the rare one that does.

Several conditions in newborns are common and aren't usually serious. Thus mothers can be more casual about them.

PHYSIOLOGIC JAUNDICE

Jaundice is a yellowish discoloration of the skin that affects all babies to some degree. It is seen more often in breast-fed babies than bottle-fed babies. Nothing needs to be done about it unless the baby is considered high risk or shows any other signs of illness.

Why do babies get jaundice?

Jaundice occurs when a yellow pigment (bilirubin) builds up in the blood. Bilirubin is normally processed in the intestinal tract and liver as foodstuffs flow freely through the gastrointestinal tract. Before birth, a mother's circulation helps the fetus clear bilirubin. After delivery the neonate must do this on his own, and it takes a little time to gear up for the task.

Why do breast-fed babies have more jaundice?

Breast-fed babies have higher bilirubin levels than formula babies because the latter get more volume and calories into their gastrointestinal tract sooner. It takes longer for a breast baby to get his gastrointestinal "circulation" going because it takes mom longer to get going. (After all, she just had a baby!)

Should I stop breast-feeding and bottle feed my baby until the jaundice goes away?

Instead of offering a bottle to get things going, it is better to offer mom and get her going. Baby will catch up quickly. Rather than decreasing breast-feeding, you should increase breast-feeding. You'd be surprised how many pediatricians still stop a healthy mother/baby pair from breast-feeding because of physiologic jaundice.

How long will the jaundice last?

Physiologic jaundice of the newborn should not persist beyond the first week of life. If it does, it should be investigated even if there are no other risk factors or signs of illness.

What makes a baby high risk?

Rather than list all the high-risk factors, it is easier to identify those babies that are low risk. Low-risk babies are born at full term after an uncomplicated pregnancy, labor, and delivery, are of normal size and healthy, and have no blood incompatibility with the mother.

How does having different blood types cause jaundice?

When blood types don't get along well, they fight. Injured and dead blood cells release their hemoglobin into the bloodstream, which the body processes into bilirubin for excretion in the urine.

I will continue to breast-feed my baby, but will formula or water help speed things up?

It is not necessary to speed things up. This is just how it is (and was before there was formula). Offering the baby formula instead of your breast will only delay your milk flow even more, and this will delay the baby's circulation from functioning to its fullest. Water may make the baby feel full and he may not want to feed.

My baby is low risk and is getting a blood test for jaundice everyday. Is this really necessary?

No. There is no need to check bilirubin levels to test for jaundice in a full-term, healthy baby born to a healthy mother.

I had some problems during pregnancy and my baby came early and was small. We're at home now, but the doctor is still checking the bilirubin everyday. Is this really necessary?

Probably. Before the baby leaves the hospital (even early discharge) blood types are checked and risk factors assessed. High-risk babies should have frequent bilirubin tests.

Are high bilirubin levels dangerous?

High bilirubin levels in *sick* infants can cause brain damage (kernicterus). Even with low levels of bilirubin kernicterus can develop in sickly newborns. However, medical care is so sophisticated today that most pediatricians have never seen or even heard of a case of kernicterus. In full-term well babies with no risk factors kernicterus will not occur even at very high bilirubin levels.

Does jaundice need to be treated with phototherapy?

Phototherapy will cause the bilirubin levels to go down, but it is doubtful that the baby is any better off.

THRUSH

Thrush is a yeast infection of the mouth acquired from the mother as the baby passes through the birth canal. White patches are visible on the cheeks, tongue, and gums. Infected infants are generally "not really sick" but may be fussy when milk or the nipple irritates the lesions. It is easily treated with antifungal medication.

My baby's tongue is white, but I thought that it was just milk. How can I tell if it is thrush or not?

Milk can easily be wiped off the tongue and thrush cannot.

My baby had thrush, but it went away with treatment. Why does it keep coming back?

Many babies with thrush also have a yeast infection in the diaper area (discrete red bumps). This should be treated with antifungal cream at the same time as the thrush. Mom's nipples and breasts may also need to be treated. Since yeast grows best in dark, wet places, both baby's bottom and mom's breasts should be "aired out" as much as possible. It is a good idea to thoroughly wash all nipples and pacifiers in warm, soapy water and keep everyone's hands clean.

GASTROESOPHAGEAL REFLUX

All babies spit up. The muscle at the junction of the stomach and esophagus is not coordinated enough to prevent stomach contents from coming back up. Some babies spit more than others, and there is no need for treatment unless the baby fails to gain weight or is sick because of it. Gastroesophageal reflux should not be confused with projectile vomiting (i.e., forcefully spewing milk across the room). You can usually decrease the amount of spitting up by trying some of the following tactics:

- Try smaller, more frequent feedings (there's less volume and pressure in the stomach).
- Do not burp your baby during or after feedings. A baby with reflux can't trap fluid much less gas. Move a full baby cautiously.
- Feed your baby in an upright position and leave her that way for 20 to 30 minutes after eating. The "C" position is not good since it leaves the junction muscle below the fluid level of the stomach.
- If you're really desperate, add 1 tablespoon of rice cereal per ounce of milk to thicken it. Just make the nipple holes larger.

CONJUNCTIVITIS

Conjunctivitis is common in newborns because the normal cleansing mechanisms of the eyes are easily clogged. This results in tearing and matting in the corners of the eyes. If your baby is otherwise well, your doctor may prescribe medication over the phone without an examination. If the baby shows any signs of illness or is at risk because of other factors or if the whites of the eyes turn red, the doctor should examine her.

My baby's tear duct gets plugged up often. My doctor said to massage the duct 10 times with my finger four times daily. Will this help?

It might help dislodge something that is currently blocking the tear duct, but I worry more about sticking your hands into the eyes of a newborn whose cleansing mechanism isn't working well. I think it is best to leave things alone and intervene only when necessary. Almost all infants outgrow this in time with or without massage. It's best to keep your hands to yourself.

CONSTIPATION

Perfectly healthy normal babies can go without a single bowel movement for up to 2 weeks. Constipation is defined as the persistent passing of pellet-sized, rock-hard stools associated with discomfort and straining. Constipation has many causes and an examination is in order. The occasional passing of hard stools or infrequent soft stools requires no medical intervention as long as the baby is well and comfortable.

Occasionally my baby is constipated and clearly uncomfortable. Isn't there anything I can do to make it easier for her to pass these hard stools?

Add a tablespoon of mineral oil to her bottle once or twice.

COLIC/CRYING

This is a tough one. Colic is defined as persistent crying for no apparent reason. Babies with colic cannot be consoled for hours, but once they finally stop, they seem perfectly okay. It is this characteristic that distinguishes the colicky baby from the sick one. It usually starts around 3 weeks of age and goes away by 3 months, although some cases last up to 6 months or so. There is no known cause or cure for colic. It makes everyone's life miserable.

How can I tell if my baby is really sick or just has colic?

At first you can't. The inconsolability of colicky babies often brings them to medical attention, but once in the doctor's office or emergency department, they are almost always smiling, happy babies. It's a good thing they are because that degree of irritability could result in admission to the hospital.

Will changing the formula or using anti-gas medications help?

Many colicky babies go through a lot of formula changes and anti-gas medications. Nothing works. (If it did, it wouldn't be colic.)

How can my doctor be sure that it's "only" colic?

A good history and physical examination can usually differentiate sick from colicky babies, but some infants undergo diagnostic tests. It's a desperate situation. As time goes by and the baby remains well except for the unrelenting crying, the diagnosis of colic is confirmed. If your baby has colic, good luck. Remember it won't last forever.

How much crying is too much?

Too much for what? A baby cannot cry itself to death. How much can you stand before you need professional reassurance that something terrible isn't wrong? If it's your first baby and it's his first or second crying jag, 15 minutes may be too much. After a few days or a couple of weeks you may be able to take 2 or 3 hours without panicking. Some colicky babies cry all the time. With time you may not get used to the crying, but you won't need professional reassurance as much.

I'm a worrywart who always thinks my baby's sick. When should I call the doctor?

Traditional signs of illness become more reliable after the first couple of months. These signs can be remembered as the three F's—fever, feeding, and fussy. Any fever, change in feeding pattern (usually loss of enthusiasm for feedings), or irritability that is not easily overcome is a sign of illness (whether it is serious or not) in a young infant. You should call your doctor to see if he needs to examine him right away or whether you should just watch him for a day or two. Keep the doctor's office posted on any changes in the three F's.

Pacifiers and Thumbsucking

Repetitive rhythmic motion such as rocking is comforting to babies. Sucking is a rhythmic repetitive motion that babies use to calm themselves. They are known to suck their thumbs in utero and make sucking motions in their sleep.

No one objects to sucking, but objections to thumbs and pacifiers abound. What are babies supposed to suck on? Well, mom, but she's not always around.

Won't a thumb or pacifier "ruin her teeth"?

The mouths of babies are very malleable. Pacifiers and thumbs may alter the shape of the mouth temporarily, but it will return to normal once these habits are discontinued. Most dentists think there's no permanent deformity unless children continue sucking past the age of 5 or 6 years. A pacifier can be taken away long before that when the baby has developed other ways to comfort himself. It's a lot harder to take away a thumb.

I hate the idea of using a pacifier to comfort my baby.

Then don't do it. If your baby calms himself without the aid of a thumb or pacifier, you are lucky. Babies given pacifiers don't suck their thumbs. Babies who are not given pacifiers suck their thumbs or go without. If your baby needs a little help (or you do!), a pacifier is a better choice than a thumb. It may take a little coaxing.

Teething

Teething is a process that begins in early infancy and persists into early adulthood. It is not an illness. The teething period coincides with the time children also tend to get mild viral illnesses, many of which go unrecognized except for fussiness. Teething is erroneously blamed for fever, runny nose, diarrhea, sleeplessness, and irritability. Although there's no doubt that an erupting tooth can cause discomfort, it is more likely that a fussy baby has a mild viral illness that does not require any treatment.

What can I do?

Teething animals chew on things. Why do you think that babies are always putting things in their mouths even when they aren't hungry? Offer a teething ring or other chewable toys. Cold ones may numb the gums for a minute or two, but the coldness on her face may be unpleasant.

5

Understanding Allergies

The immune system acts as the body's security force, keeping out intruders that don't belong and restraining natives that get out of line. When it works well, the immune system protects us from infection and cancer. When it works too well and attacks when it shouldn't, we suffer from allergies.

Allergic symptoms are the result of an overactive or hypersensitive immune system. The body is desperately trying to rid itself of irritants (allergens) by washing them away and preventing reentry. This accounts for swollen and runny eyes, congested and runny noses, and tight, congested lungs as well as bouts of coughing and sneezing. The skin responds by itching so the allergen can be removed by scratching.

A person is not born allergic but rather with a tendency to become allergic. An allergic person becomes sensitive to substances in the environment. It's not just a coincidence that he was born in exactly the wrong place. No matter where he lives, sooner or later he will react to his surroundings. It usually takes years to develop significant allergic symptoms so infants are generally spared for a couple of years.

Allergic tendencies run in families. The "target organs" (eyes, nose, lungs, and skin) may vary from one family member to another and may even vary in the same allergic individual. With the exception of steroids, which incapacitate the entire immune system, there is no single medication that will treat all allergic symptoms. The types of medications used depend on which target organs are symptomatic. Many research efforts are focused on finding out which parts of the immune system are responsible for hypersensitivity reactions. The future holds promise for allergy sufferers.

This chapter will also clarify some misconceptions about food allergies, insect bites, and penicillin allergy.

Allergic Rhinitis

Allergic rhinitis is caused by allergens that irritate the nasal lining. It results in sneezing, dilation of the blood vessels in the nose (congestion), and the release of fluid—all with the goal of washing out the irritant and keeping it from reentering. Symptoms last as long as the irritant is in the environment. If the nose is the only target organ, the patient doesn't feel too bad.

What are some of the common allergens?

Everyone knows about pollens, weeds, and grasses, but cockroaches, dust mites, molds, and cats are some of the worst offenders.

I can never tell if my daughter has a cold or an allergy. Any suggestions?

It is often difficult to tell if young children have a cold or allergy. A cold virus will elicit the same response as an allergen when it enters the nose, even though the processes are biochemically different. Generally a child with a cold feels "bad all over." Colds are more common in the colder months when children are in close contact inside. Allergies are more common in the spring and fall when children are outside a lot. As the child gets older, typical patterns develop and you can usually tell whether she has a cold or allergy. Many times a child has both.

But what if her drainage is thick and green?

Let's straighten this out once and for all. Noses are not sterile. Germs are always present, but the immune system keeps the numbers down and the child isn't infected. When the immune system is busy reacting to a cold virus or allergen, the bacterial count in the nose increases. The mucus thickens and turns green. As soon as the cold resolves (usually around 7 to 10 days) or the allergen has disappeared, the bacterial count returns to normal and the thick, green mucus clears up. This is the natural course of a cold or allergic reaction.

What if the green, runny nose doesn't clear up?

Complications do occur, especially in children who have small airways and openings that cannot drain well. Over-the-counter cold formulas can lead to complications by interfering with the body's protective mechanisms. If the thick, green mucus persists beyond 10 to 14 days and the child's general condition is deteriorating rather than improving, she should be examined for complications. Most children will still recover uneventfully without antibiotics, but at this point a few doses of antibiotics may speed things up. Just remember that casual antibiotic use has its own list of complications.

What's the best treatment for my daughter's allergies?
Traditionally, allergic rhinitis is treated systemically with oral antihistamines. Steroid sprays, which have served adults well, have been used more frequently in children in the past couple of years. Another option is the *prevention* of symptoms with daily use of the nonsteroidal nasal spray cromolyn.

What about decongestants?
Systemic oral decongestants do not work well, and topical decongestants must be used cautiously because allergic rhinitis can persist for weeks and the spray can only be used for a couple of days. Since allergies are chronic and lifelong, it might be best to reserve treatment for the days when a child feels bad and not just when she has a runny nose.

My doctor gave me a new nasal spray for my allergies and it's not a steroid or decongestant. Would that help my daughter?
Two recently approved nasal sprays for adults (azelastine and ipratropium) may be useful in children. Both can relieve the runny nose due to allergy and ipratropium can even relieve the runny nose from a cold.

Are you saying that this new medication can stop the runny nose from a cold? That's great! Where can I get some?
It's not that great. The nasal spray has to be used every 4 hours and with each subsequent dose its effects are shorter lived. Since you can expect the runny nose from a cold or allergy to last 1 to 2 weeks, the medication is not practical in most instances. My experience shows that most children can only tolerate a couple of doses before their nose becomes too dry and they experience an uncomfortable burning sensation. As soon as the dose wears off, the runny nose returns.

Oh. So why bother?
Ipratropium nasal spray my be useful at naptime or bedtime or for a special occasion such as a birthday party.

When should my child see an allergist?
If your child has allergic symptoms severe enough to result in frequent complications (ear infections, sinusitis, lots of missed day care or school,

sleeplessness poor growth, or asthma) that cannot be controlled with any of the available medications, she should see the allergist for skin testing. The results of these tests may suggest that additional enviornmental control measures would be helpful or may lead to a decision to begin immunotherapy (allergy shots). If you have tried all the environmental control measures you can tolerate and you have no intention of proceeding with skin testing and allergy shots, the allergist doesn't have anything to contribute.

When can I have skin testing done?

It can be done at any age, but the younger the patient, the more likely the results will be misleading. For instance, if a young child reacts, she most likely is allergic; but if she doesn't, an allergy can't be ruled out. Fortunately, it takes years to develop significant allergic symptoms, and the question of allergy testing rarely arises before the age of 3 years or so. By then testing is fairly reliable in experienced hands.

We've done the skin testing and now know what to avoid. My daughter is going to feel better now, right?

Maybe. Allergen avoidance is ideal, but in most cases it is impossible. Tossing out the cat and most of the toys, avoiding cigarette smoke, keeping the house dust free, sealing off the basement, eliminating all cockroaches and dust mites, staying indoors, staying outdoors, and buying expensive air filters, dehumidifiers, and linens may be all you need to do to get significant relief.

Can't I just keep the cat outside?

It's best to give the cat away and move. Cat dander stays suspended in the air for a long time before it settles down on every thing; it is then easily resuspended in the air when someone walks through. Cat allergens linger long after the cat has gone.

Do allergy shots work?

Immunotherapy with allergy shots can make a significant difference if you can make the long-term commitment (2 to 3 years) to follow the treatment plan. With careful skin testing, allergy shot preparation, and strict adherence to the injection schedule, allergy shots can work, especially for inhaled allergens such as dust mites, pollen, and cats. It is less effective for molds and doesn't work at all for foods. Environmental controls still need to be continued as tolerated.

Allergic Conjunctivitis

Allergic conjunctivitis is just like its counterpart allergic rhinitis. The eyes swell and tear in response to an allergen in an attempt to rid itself of the offender. Most people with allergic conjunctivitis also have allergic rhinitis. Treatment consists of systemic or topical antihistamines or topical non-steroidal anti-inflammatory drops (cromolyn and others). Topical steroid drops are not recommended for allergic conjunctivitis because of potentially serious complications. As is the case for allergic rhinitis, topical decongestants are not recommended. They may get the red out for a few hours, but the allergic process can last for days or weeks. Washing the eyes out frequently with sterile saline eyedrops can offer significant relief if your child will cooperate.

How do I know if my child's pinkeye is an allergic reaction or an infection?

Allergic conjunctivitis can be difficult to differentiate from viral or bacterial conjunctivitis in young children. The discharge from allergic conjunctivitis should be clear, but just as in the case of the nose, it is just a matter of a day or two before it thickens up and turns green. However, it is more common in young children for allergic eyes to become secondarily infected because of their tendency to rub their itchy eyes after wiping their runny noses. I almost always treat these children with topical antibiotic eyedrops and instruct them to keep their hands clean and away from their faces. Clean hands and sterile saline eyewashes are all that are needed for older cooperative kids, even though many parents insist on antibiotic drops.

Asthma or Reactive Airway Disease

Asthma is the lung counterpart of allergic disease. Most children with asthma will also have allergic rhinitis, and the many irritants that provoke the nose will also provoke the lungs. This is variable, however, for asthma is known for its unpredictable manifestations even in the same individual.

Asthma is characterized by wheezing and/or coughing in response to anything the lungs perceive as irritating. In addition to the usual list of irritants, asthmatics can react to foods, low humidity, low temperatures, cold viruses, stress, exercise, or wind. The lungs of some asthmatics can be as reliable as a barometer for detecting weather changes. It is not a psychological disease, but frequent shortness of breath, loss of sleep, and medication can have a dramatic impact on the psyche.

What exactly is wheezing?

Contrary to popular belief, wheezing is subtle. It is a very quiet whistling sound (usually only detectable with a stethoscope) caused by partial obstruction of the smaller airways of the lungs. In view of the coughing, crying, grunting, crouping, gurgling, etc. that are characteristic of sick children, it takes a lot of practice, a good stethoscope, and patience to detect wheezing in young children. Even in older kids it can be difficult without their cooperation.

So that noisy, congested breathing that I can hear from the other room is not wheezing?

No, it's not. Louder breathing comes from higher up in the airway. A quieter sound comes from lower in the airway. It makes sense if you think about it.

So you're saying that my son's *deep, loud* cough isn't coming from his chest at all?

That's right, it's not.

Then how am I supposed to know if my son is wheezing or not?

No one expects you to know when your son is wheezing, but if he is a wheezer, in time both you and he will learn to recognize other more obvious signs that suggest that wheezing is present even if you aren't able to hear it. The most obvious is the presence of a *pattern* of cough, especially an unrelenting nighttime cough that lasts throughout the night with no intervening quiet periods. With experience, you will be able to tell just by the way the cough sounds. There are some other signs such as shallow, rapid breathing and sinking in of the chest during breathing that you will also learn to recognize.

My kid coughs all the time but my doctor has told me many times that he is not asthmatic and not to worry. How can he be so sure?

Kids generally cough in response to a tickle in the throat caused by postnasal drip. This is not asthma and will not respond to asthma medications. Your doctor is probably correct. However, if your child or other family members have any additional signs of allergy or asthma (such as postnasal drip), a more careful history and physical examination may suggest the possibility of reactive airway disease or asthma. Sometimes a nighttime cough may be the only manifestation of asthma, but a closer look will usually reveal other indications of allergic disease.

Okay, so he might have a "little asthma." Since most of his coughs will usually be caused by postnasal drip, how can I know when to start my son's asthma medicine?

Good question. If he's never had any significant discomfort from asthma or cough, it is reasonable to wait until you know for sure if he is wheezing before starting his asthma treatments. If his asthma has caused him significant problems in the past, it is best to start him on his asthma medicines as soon as he has any allergic or cold symptoms, including postnasal drip. It is important to remember that the same irritants that trigger nasal, throat, and eye symptoms can also trigger the lungs. Be alert to these early warnings and get him on his asthma medicine before he has a chance to develop potentially serious chest symptoms.

What if he only coughs when he runs or when the weather is cold?

Some asthmatics only wheeze (or cough or feel chest tightness) when they exercise or when the barometer drops or the air is cold or dry. Reactive airways are very peculiar indeed.

What's the difference between asthma, reactive airway disease, and bronchitis?

I'm so glad you asked. In children these terms all signify the same thing. Before good asthma drugs were available, asthmatics were stereotypically pale, sickly, skinny kids (i.e., "wimps"). With a better understanding of the illness and the availability of effective medications and treatments, this is no longer the case (in fact, it seems to be a prerequisite to being on the Olympic team). Unfortunately, the stereotype still prevails in the minds of many parents. They shudder at the mention of "asthma" but have no problem with "reactive airway disease." "Bronchitis" and "walking pneumonia" are common terms used casually by doctors when they mistakenly blame lung symptoms on infection rather than allergy.

I don't want "asthma" on my child's medical record. Can you just put "reactive airway disease," "bronchitis," or "pneumonia"?

The insurance companies aren't fooled that easily. They know asthma when they see it. It is very unusual for a healthy child to get a single case of pneumonia, much less several in the first few years of life. "A rose is a rose. . . . "

My physician has always treated all my children's bouts of bronchitis with antibiotics. Are you saying that their wheezing wasn't due to infection, but allergy?

Most likely. Allergies are very common and by definition are recurrent. Lung infections are unusual, and when they do occur, they are almost always viral in origin and antibiotics are ineffective. The first or second wheezing episodes can optimistically be attributed to infectious bad luck, but more than that takes a lot of imagination. There's a saying in pediatrics that goes, "If it wheezes, it doesn't need antibiotics."

My doctor treats my son's asthma with albuterol, antihistamines, and sometimes steroids but also often prescribes an antibiotic as well. Is that okay?

Like allergic rhinitis, asthma is not usually associated with a bacterial infectious process. However, in certain situations antibiotics may be indicated. If the bronchoconstriction and mucous plugging are persistent, there is increased risk of a secondary bacterial infection. As time goes by the patient's condition deteriorates despite optimal treatment. Sometimes a patient will just not improve, and bacterial overgrowth may be playing a role. In addition, untreated bacterial sinusitis can trigger or aggravate asthma. Most doctors will give an antibiotic to an asthmatic whose condition is deteriorating or is not responding to other supportive measures.

Why are asthmatic symptoms so variable?

No one knows. Asthma never really goes away, and even when an asthmatic is symptom free, careful testing shows that the lungs are still hypersensitive. It may have to do with the body's inability to have "all systems on go." A letdown in immune surveillance for whatever reason benefits the asthmatic.

What is the best treatment for asthma?

There are as many treatment regimens for asthma as there are asthmatics since the disease is so variable even in the same individual. The mainstay of treatment is bronchodilator therapy with albuterol (Ventolin or Proventil). This medication works best when inhaled into the lungs via a nebulizer or hand-held cannister (metered-dose inhaler), but it can be given as a liquid to small children. Any asthmatic old enough to swallow a pill should be on inhalation therapy instead.

In addition, asthmatics can be treated with inhaled or oral steroids and antihistamines. Inhaled nonsteroidal anti-inflammatory agents (cromolyn) can be used several times daily for prevention, but they have no effect during an ongoing attack. Concomitant treatment of allergic rhinitis is also beneficial. Fluids keep the mucus thin and easier to mobilize.

Is there something besides medication that will help?

Because of the potential seriousness of the symptoms, allergen avoidance and immunotherapy are more important for the asthmatic than someone who only has allergic rhinitis or conjunctivitis. It is a good idea for most asthmatics to see an allergist periodically. Since there is so much variability in the course of the disease even in the same patient, treatment must be individualized. However, there is no question that exposure to tobacco smoke should be avoided and a yearly influenza vaccination given.

My baby wheezed a couple of months ago. Does he have asthma?

It's too early to tell. Asthma is defined as recurrent wheezing (or sometimes just coughing). If he wheezes again and again, then he probably does. Some infants will get a viral infection (respiratory syncytial virus [RSV] bronchiolitis) that provokes wheezing during their first year of life. This is considered a one-time event and does not constitute asthma. However, many infants and young children become infected with RSV without developing wheezing, presumably because they were not born with reactive airway disease or their illness was milder for whatever reason. It is not a good sign that your baby has already had a wheezing episode, but it does not necessarily mean that he will become an asthmatic.

My baby had RSV bronchiolitis when he was 6 months old. He wheezes all the time now. Is that what caused it?

Maybe, maybe not. It is the chicken and egg thing. Was your baby *born* to be a wheezer and RSV was the first in a long line of irritants to elicit the asthmatic response or did the RSV cause his lungs to become hypersensitive and wheezy from then on? This is a very hot topic these days. If RSV infection early in life could be prevented (e.g., by vaccination), would we see a decrease in the incidence of asthma? Some experts think so. Remember, asthma runs in families, but so does the ability to resist infection.

Do I need to give my asthmatic baby albuterol every time he gets a cold, cough, or wheezing spell?

Not necessarily. Although there is a possibility that your child could have a serious asthma attack, it is unusual in young babies (the immune system isn't "mature" enough yet). Most infants are very tolerant of wheezing. Keep in mind that albuterol can make kids irritable and hyperactive. It is frequently a judgment call whether to treat an infant with oral or inhaled bronchodilator therapy.

Any infant with noticeable respiratory distress needs to be seen by a pediatrician for evaluation and treatment. If infants are happy and playful and sleeping and eating well, most of the time they do not need to be treated at all but only carefully observed for signs of deterioration.

Should I have a pulmonologist or allergist see my asthmatic child?

Since asthma is a chronic and potentially life-threatening disease, it is a good idea to have another doctor familiar with your child's condition. Although most cases of asthma are routine and easily handled in a pediatrician's office, more intensive therapy and monitoring may be necessary in severe cases. An occasional routine checkup by a specialist to keep him updated on your child's condition is a good idea in the event that you need him in an emergency.

Will my son outgrow his asthma?

The course of asthma is extremely variable and unpredictable, but most children seem to eventually outgrow it. However, some remnants return occasionally.

Allergic Skin, Sensitive Skin, or Atopic Dermatitis and Food Allergy

Atopic dermatitis is the skin counterpart of allergic disease. Atopic, hypersensitive, or allergic skin tends to be very dry and easily irritated for no apparent reason. It itches a lot. Like the other allergic diseases, atopic dermatitis is chronic and treatment is aimed at reducing symptoms to a tolerable level. It does seem to improve somewhat as children get older. Food allergy, of course, is an important component of atopic dermatitis.

My baby's skin is very dry and sensitive. Does he have atopic dermatitis?

Infants can show signs of atopic dermatitis such as red, dry, scaling patches of skin on their cheeks at a very early age. They are also prone to other rashes and are sensitive to every thing. They are usually irritable, probably because of the itching.

That sounds like what he has. Would baby lotion help?

An understandable, but frequent mistake is overbathing and applying various lotions and creams to moisturize and help clear up the problem. This invariably makes the situation worse and sets up a vicious cycle.

What should I do? His skin looks bad and I know he doesn't feel well.

Treatment of atopic dermatitis includes the following measures:

1. Avoid overbathing. Atopic skin is lacking an adequate protective layer, making it very dry and easily irritated. It is best not to disturb what little natural protection atopic skin has. Only wash off obviously dirty spots with Dove soap and warm water. A 5-minute bath in a few inches of water or a quick shower every couple of days is sufficient.

2. Apply emollients liberally to seal in natural oils and keep out irritants. I like Vaseline petrolatum jelly because it is oil based rather than water based and won't evaporate and take moisture with it. A less messy alternative is Eucerin. Some dermatologists recommend Crisco.

3. Use 1% hydrocortisone cream sparingly for red, irritated areas on the face. Get by with as little as possible for as short a time as possible.

4. Use a medium-potency steroid cream sparingly on red, irritated skin on the body. Again, use as little as possible for as short a period of time as possible.

5. Use systemic antihistamines such as Benadryl to control itching. Some experts believe that all the lesions of atopic dermatitis are caused by scratching. Thus, if you stop the scratching, the skin will clear up.

6. Treat breaks in the skin or refractory lesions with systemic anti-staphylococcal antibiotics such as erythromycin. Other experts believe that individuals with atopic dermatitis are only allergic to staphylococcal ("staph") bacteria and controlling the bacterial count will eliminate atopic dermatitis. Remember not to mix the newer antihistamines such as Seldane and Hismanal with erythromycins such as Biaxin.

7. Do not use oral steroids. Atopic dermatitis is chronic, and the risks of long-term or frequent intermittent steroid use outweigh the temporary benefits.

What causes atopic dermatitis?

Atopic dermatitis is one of the most frustrating illnesses that children, pediatricians, and parents have to deal with. Like all other allergic diseases, there is a strong genetic component. No one knows what triggers atopic dermatitis, but food may play a larger role than in other allergic diseases. It is reasonable to try to eliminate known allergens such as milk or eggs from the diet of those infants with severe, unremitting problems, but most attempts to do this are unsuccessful in clearing up the skin. Formula changes may sometimes help, especially when formula constitutes the entire diet. Like other allergic diseases, the course of atopic dermatitis is chronic, variable, and unpredictable.

I am breast-feeding my baby. Can what I eat cause my baby's skin problems?

Maybe. Some experts think that babies can "be sensitized" through breast-feeding because of foods their moms have consumed. However, evidence shows that prolonged and exclusive breast-feeding decreases the incidence of atopic skin problems in infants. There is also evidence that fetuses can be sensitized to foods in utero. If there is a family history of atopic dermatitits, it would be a good idea to consult an allergist and consider limiting your diet from early pregnancy until your infant is weaned.

Which foods are most likely to cause problems?

The most common foods that elicit allergy are:

Milk	Seafood	Berries
Eggs	Soybeans	Wheat
Nuts		

New foods should be carefully introduced one at a time into a baby's diet. However, special caution should be taken with the foods listed above, especially if there is a family history of allergy.

Is it too late to watch what I eat and what I offer my baby to eat?

No. Even though your baby may already be sensitized, eliminating suspect foods from his diet may help clear his skin. Remember that food is only one possible trigger of atopic dermatitis.

I know a lot of people with food allergies, but I don't know any with atopic dermatitis. How's that?

Food *intolerance* is often confused with food allergy, and data suggest that only about 5% of the population has a food allergy. Of this percentage, only some will manifest atopic dermatitis.

What's the difference?

A food allergy is an immunologic reaction to a food that can be life threatening and can be manifested by gastrointestinal tract, respiratory tract, and most commonly skin symptoms. Food intolerance is not immunologically mediated, and symptoms are mild and usually restricted to the gastrointestinal tract. *Any* amount of an offensive food can result in life-threatening allergic reactions, but the reaction caused by food intolerance is usually dose dependent.

What should I look for when introducing a new food?

Atopic dermatitis or hives is usually the first sign of food allergy in children, but gastrointestinal symptoms such as diarrhea, vomiting, gas, and bloating are sometimes the first indication. Life-threatening respiratory problems are the first symptoms seen in the most severe cases.

Is there any treatment for food allergy?

Specific treatment should be handled by an allergist, but incomplete avoidance of the offensive food is required. Since foods have so many "disguised" ingredients, a dietician may need to be consulted. Food allergy is considered a lifelong condition, and immunotherapy does not work. If a child has a history of a severe food allergy, an EpiPen should be readily available for injection in emergency situations.

How do you diagnose a food allergy?

The best way to diagnose a food allergy is by careful history taking. Skin testing for food allergy is not as reliable as for other allergens and should be performed only when the history strongly suggests there is a problem. If the skin test is negative, it is likely that the child can eat the food safely, but a positive skin test is not necessarily conclusive. A positive skin test is only meaningful if the clinical history suggests an allergy.

My son gets severe stomach cramps, gas, and diarrhea when he drinks milk. Is he allergic?

Probably not allergic, but he may be lactose intolerant. Many people have decreased levels of the enzyme lactase in their intestinal tracts and are unable to break down the sugar (lactose) found in cow's milk. The undigested lactose causes the abdominal symptoms. Most lactose-intolerant people can digest *some* milk (i.e., they are not totally deficient in the enzyme) without any problem or with only mild symptoms. Lactase levels can decrease with age (higher levels in infancy and childhood, lower levels in adults) and are genetically determined. Lactase levels can also decrease temporarily after a *prolonged* bout of diarrhea.

My daughter became swollen and turned red after she ate peanut butter. Is she allergic?

Most likely and it would be wise to eliminate all peanut products completely and forever. It would also be a good idea to see a dietician and an allergist.

My 15-month-old daughter just developed hives. She's had several new foods in the past couple of days. How do I know which is responsible?

You probably won't be able to figure this out unless it happens again and there is clearly only one suspect the second time. There are many other causes of hives besides foods. Since it was only a rash and she has had no previous food reactions, a cautious approach is recommended. If you suspect she has had other reactions or if she had any other associated symptoms in addition to the rash, you should see an allergist.

Insect Bites and Stings

Everyone will have some local reactions to an insect bite or sting since the skin has been penetrated. Depending on the amount of venom injected and the trauma to the skin, local reactions at the site may range from a pinhead-sized bump to a red, hard lesion the size of a half-dollar. It may take a day or two for the local reaction to peak before it starts to subside. Scratching and rubbing will exaggerate the local inflammatory response.

In patients with an allergic response to the insect venom there may be skin reactions distant from the site as well as systemic symptoms that can be life threatening. Insects belonging to the Hymenoptera class (wasps, honey bees, yellow jackets, hornets, and fire ants) are the most likely to elicit allergic responses. Allergic patients should wear protective clothing, be vigilant, and carry an EpiPen if there is a chance they will be exposed. They should see an allergist and consider desensitizing injections.

My son is not allergic, but bites and stings cause a big, red itchy spot. Why?

Isolated, discrete, circumscribed lesions are local reactions to the trauma or venom. Even if they are big, red, and itchy, they are not infected or allergic. Applying 1% hydrocortisone cream (Cortaid) will decrease the inflammatory response and the itching in the first couple of days after a bite or sting. Benadryl cream can also help but will probably not be as effective as 1% hydrocortisone cream.

How can I prevent these lesions from getting infected?

Clean hands, short nails, and soap and water along with 1% hydrocortisone cream to decrease the itching usually can prevent the onset of infection.

How do I know if the bites are infected or not?

An infection will not develop for a week or so. If scratching continues for a week after being bitten and the lesions never seem to heal, there is probably an infection. Washing the bites several times daily with soap and water, keeping the child's hands clean and nails short, and using 1% hydrocortisone cream or Benadryl to stop the itching may avoid the need for antibiotics. Cover the bites with a gauze if it won't get too dirty. If the lesions don't start clearing up within 24 to 48 hours, you probably need to see the doctor.

My son stepped in an ant pile and his entire lower leg is swollen and red. What should I do?

Multiple bites are no different except that the individual local reactions may coalesce, resulting in larger areas of redness and swelling that may look like infection although it is not. It still takes time for infection to develop.

The treatment remains the same except, depending on the extent of the area, oral Benadryl may make more sense than topical treatment. Oral steroids are generally not necessary since the inflammatory response has already peaked by the time medical care is sought. It just takes time for the swelling to resolve. In rare cases these larger lesions may represent a mild allergic reaction and oral steroids may be indicated. It can be a warning of more serious reactions in the future and caution is advised.

Penicillin Allergy

Most people who think that they are allergic to penicillin really are not, but a doctor would be crazy to prescribe it to someone who says he's allergic to it. Penicillin and its related drugs amoxicillin and Augmentin are very useful in pediatric medicine, and it's unfortunate to be restricted in prescribing them because people erroneously think they are allergic.

However, penicillin allergy cannot be easily dismissed since it can be life threatening. In infants and young children the "reaction" is frequently just a symptom of the illness itself (e.g., rash or vomiting). It is best to determine if a reaction is allergic or not at the time it occurs and note it in the chart.

Does penicillin allergy run in families?

Penicillin allergy, like all other allergies, does run in families. This can be helpful in determining if a reaction is allergic, but a positive family history in itself should not preclude its use if a child clearly needs it. If a parent strongly objects because of a bad personal experience with penicillin, obviously this cannot be ignored.

How can you tell if a reaction is a side effect or an allergic reaction?

Physicians may have difficulty in deciding if a penicillin reaction is an allergic response or just a side effect. The problem most commonly arises in infants who break out in a rash when they are on amoxicillin. The "penicillin allergic" label then follows them through life unnecessarily.

A typical scenario is as follows:

Jack is 8 months old and started running a temperature on Saturday night. He was irritable and didn't eat or sleep well. On Sunday he seemed better, played a little, and drank his bottle. Sunday night he had a temperature of 104° F. In the office on Monday Jack's temperature was 101° F, but the pediatrician could not find any source of the fever. A wait and see course was taken since he seemed to be holding his own. By Wednesday Jack still had a fever and mom was worried. The doctor checked him again, ran some tests, and found nothing except a "little redness" of his eardrums. Jack's mom was given a prescription for amoxicillin for his ear infection. Jack was given two doses on Wednesday. His fever finally broke Wednesday night and mom and the doctor were relieved. That amoxicillin was good stuff!

Thursday morning Jack feels fine except that his body is covered with a rash. Mom calls the pediatrician's office and this is when the confusion begins. The busy doctor communicating via the office nurse comes to one of two possible conclusions:

Conclusion 1: Jack has roseola, a common viral infection in infants. It is characterized by 4 or 5 days of high temperature with no obvious source of infection followed by resolution of the fever and subsequent appearance of a rash. The diagnosis is made retrospectively when Jack is already recovering.

Conclusion 2: Jack is allergic to amoxicillin and needs a different antibiotic for his ear infection. The rash broke out after two or three doses of amoxicillin for "early ear infection." Amoxicillin seemingly worked well for Jack except that he's now tagged as "allergic to amoxicillin" and can never get it again. He has also been switched to a second antibiotic to finish out his 10-day course. In addition, Jack now "gets ear infections." This scenario can repeat itself whenever he gets a fever. Eventually there could be a whole list of antibiotics that Jack is "allergic to," "can't tolerate," or "don't work."

Unfortunately, this little drama is all too common. If there is any doubt, the "penicillin allergic" label must be attached. If there is a special need for penicillin, an allergist can perform specific tests to diagnose an allergy and administer desensitizing injections if necessary.

6

Common Childhood Diseases and Problems

Upper Respiratory Infections (Colds)

There are about 200 different viruses that cause colds. Healthy children can average five to eight colds a year. Cold viruses are caught from other people; your child doesn't get a cold from cold weather, wet hair, or barefeet (sorry, mom).

Why are colds so much more common than other viral illnesses?

Colds are just a constellation of symptoms that together prevent a virus from entering the body and causing disease. The mouth, throat, and nose are only the portals of entry. (Stomach viruses are the next most common illnesses.)

I always hear that a cold just has to "runs its course." What does that mean anyway?

A cold lasts approximately 7 to 10 days and medications will not alter its course. Infants and young children may have a high temperature the first 2 to 3 days. They are irritable and have a sore throat, their appetite decreases, and they will frequently awaken at night because of difficulty in breathing through the nose or coughing. The mucus in the nose will turn green by the third or fourth day, but this will begin to resolve by the seventh to tenth day. The cough may last a couple of weeks.

What if the symptoms aren't better by then?

There are hundreds of viruses that cause colds, and some naturally last a little longer than others. If the symptoms of a cold persist beyond 10 days, it could signal a complication such as an ear infection or sinusitis in a *deteriorating* child.

I worry that it might turn into pneumonia?

Bad colds do not "turn into" pneumonia. Colds are caused by viruses, and although pneumonia is also caused by viruses, they are usually not the same ones. A cold virus will cause a cold and a pneumonia virus will cause pneumonia. It just takes longer for the lung symptoms to become manifest, giving the impression that the cold has turned into pneumonia.

My daughter caught double pneumonia after a really bad cold. She had to be hospitalized and get antibiotics. How can I prevent this from happening again?

Bacteria cause about 10% of the cases of pneumonia. When this occurs, it is commonly after a prolonged viral illness such as a bad cold, influenza, or chickenpox. Bacteria that are normally easily warded off by an intact immune system can prevail when a person is in a weakened state. This is a nonpreventable secondary infection. It is diagnosed fairly easily because these children suddenly deteriorate at a time when rapid recovery is expected. As long as the fever doesn't return and the child's overall condition is not deteriorating, it is unlikely that there is a secondary bacterial pneumonia.

How can I tell if it's a cold or an allergy?

Early cold symptoms can be confused with allergic symptoms, especially in younger children. A cold displays a typical pattern of worsening over 3 to 4 days and then improving. It is more likely to be associated with fever, decreased appetite, and general irritability and fatigue. Allergies tend to run in families and are seasonal. Allergic symptoms can last for weeks with little variation from day to day.

There are so many cold medicines for children. Which one should I buy?

Cold formulas have many side effects and do not counteract the body's defense mechanisms against viral invasion (thank goodness). Tylenol at naptime or bedtime may help relieve general discomfort temporarily.

What about those new zinc lozenges?

The initial data indicate that frequent use of zinc lozenges within the first 24 hours of the onset of cold symptoms may significantly decrease the discomfort of a cold. So far they seem harmless and may prove to be an important breakthrough in cold therapy, but studies have not been completed at this writing and no confirmatory studies have been undertaken.

What about that herb *Echinaceae* or whatever?

I am not an expert on herbal medicine, but I do recognize that wild plants are a source for many important medicines. However, plants are made up of many substances that may have pharmacologic effects, some of which may be harmful. I worry about purity, proper dosing, side effects, and proper preparation. Since *Echinaceae* is considered a food, it is not subjected to the same kind of scrutiny and regulation that approved drugs are. It is such an inexact science with so many variables that I wouldn't consider using it for my own kids. Fortunately, the drug companies do take heed to the herbalists' claims and eventually market the product if it proves safe and effective.

I feel just awful when my baby suffers from a cold. Isn't there anything else I can do?

It's good to remember that you feel worse than your baby does and that the more battles fought in childhood the fewer battles will have to be fought as an adult. Building immunity is as much a task in infancy and childhood as growing and learning to walk.

What do you do when *your* kids have colds?

Good question. I think of it as an immunologic exercise. As hard as it is, I try my best to do nothing. I offer them lots of special privileges: cokes, popsicles, ice cream, TV, my bed! I make sure they get lots of fluids. If a sore throat is causing them discomfort, I give them Life Savers or Luden's cough drops (they like wild cherry) because they taste good and keep their throat wet. Occasionally I resort to Tylenol or Motrin for particularly miserable days. At bedtime I frequently break down and drug them with Benadryl for its sedative and cough-suppressing properties. (Sometimes I take it instead!) I put a tall glass of ice-cold water and a box of Kleenex by their beds. When they're older, I will try Afrin nasal spray, and for unremitting coughs, codeine.

Influenza

Influenza is a moderate to severe illness caused by members of the influenza virus family. There are two major types, A and B. Influenza is epidemic in the cold weather months. It is primarily a respiratory illness involving the lungs, but it can affect the upper airways as well. It is characterized by fever lasting up to 10 to 12 days, cough and chest discomfort, fatigue, and generalized aches. It can take 2 to 3 weeks to recover. Most healthy people who contract influenza do not develop serious complications, but high-risk patients such as young infants and those with lung or heart disease can die from complications.

I thought "flu" was vomiting and diarrhea. Is that true?

Diarrhea and vomiting due to gastrointestinal viruses and bad colds are also commonly referred to as "flu" or "24-hour flu," but these have no relation to the viruses that cause influenza.

What's a "flu shot"?

A vaccine is developed each year that incorporates the three strains of flu virus that are most likely to circulate. A yearly vaccine is the best way to avoid the symptoms of influenza. Almost anyone over the age of 6 months can be immunized.

I've heard that a flu shot can actually give you the flu. Why take that chance?

Influenza vaccine is a killed virus and cannot result in infection, but like all vaccines it can cause some mild local symptoms such as arm soreness. It takes 2 to 4 weeks for the vaccine to provide protection, and since influenza season coincides with the cold season, many people mistakenly believe that their influenza vaccine made them ill.

Does it work?

It is no better or worse than the "routine" vaccines that you are familiar with. No vaccine is perfect, but immunized persons who do become infected will have much milder symptoms than had they not been immunized.

How many flu shots do my kids need?

The first year they need two shots, one month apart. After the first year one shot is sufficient.

Isn't there a cure for flu now?

We can treat influenza A, but not influenza B, and only if started within the first 24 hours of the onset of symptoms. Both A and B strains can circulate every year.

Can influenza be prevented with medication?

Influenza A can be prevented with Flumadine when taken daily during the flu season. It is a reasonable choice for the 2- to 4-week period before the vaccination "kicks in." Medication can also be offered to family members if influenza occurs in the household.

Croup

Croup is a viral infection of the airway that involves the larynx (voicebox), trachea (windpipe), and bronchi (major airways of the lung). In young children these airways are relatively small, and when they become inflamed from a viral infection, there is increased resistance to airflow. This accounts for the loud, noisy breathing and croupy cough. Smaller children are more apt to have significant respiratory distress than larger children simply because their airways are smaller.

The illness runs its course in 7 to 10 days, peaking in severity around day 4. Frequently the child has a high fever the first 2 to 3 days and a runny nose. Symptoms are generally worse at night. A croupy infant needs a lot of extra tender loving care and fluids. Most infants do well without any medical intervention.

My baby sounds terrible. How do I know if she's doing okay or not?

Your baby is doing fine if she's taking fluids well even if she won't eat, she has playful periods, and she's attentive to her environment and not preoccupied with her own breathing.

Should I use a cool or warm mist?

Babies with croup breathe fast and do not take fluids well, which can "dry out" the airways, especially in the cold months when croup is most common and the heat is on. A mist can offer some relief for the irritated airways. It is the hydration, not the temperature that is important, but there are so many reports of parents and siblings getting burned that cool mist is preferable.

If humidifiers and vaporizers are not cleaned daily according to the manufacturer's recommendations, they may cause more harm than good. If you're not inclined to do this, don't use them.

When should I worry?

Call the doctor if her breathing is so labored that she cannot take fluids, she cannot be distracted by playing or any other activity, and she cannot rest.

If she is in respiratory distress, what will happen?

More seriously ill infants can be given an injection of steroids in the pediatrician's office or the emergency department to decrease the inflammation in the airways and make breathing easier. Occasionally an infant must be treated in the emergency department or hospitalized for oxygen, intravenous fluids, and other medications.

Pneumonia

Pneumonia is an infection of the lungs of viral or bacterial origin. Most children with pneumonia are really sick. They don't eat or play, are irritable and listless, and are not interested in their surroundings.

Although the early symptoms of pneumonia may be similar to those of a common cold (runny nose, fever, and cough—the defense mechanisms), pneumonia is an infection of the lungs from the outset, whether caused by a virus or bacterium. The viruses that cause bad colds do not "turn into" pneumonia, but they can weaken the immune system and permit a secondary bacterial invasion.

What's the difference between viral and bacterial pneumonias?

Approximately 90% of all pneumonias are viral and involve both lungs diffusely as well as the upper respiratory system (nose and throat). Viral pneumonia is equivalent to a cold in the head and chest. It is characterized by fever, runny nose, and frequently wheezing. It is associated with a continuous cough, both day and night, which can persist for weeks. Children feel bad. Except for pneumonia caused by the influenza virus, the course of viral pneumonia cannot be altered by medication. Wheezing may respond to bronchodilator therapy with albuterol. Symptoms improve within a week or so, although the cough may last for several weeks.

Bacterial pneumonia is uncommon in healthy children. It is usually localized to one or maybe two lobes of one lung, and associated upper respiratory symptoms are not prominent. Children with pneumonia have a fever and feel bad; older children frequently can point to a painful place in their chest. There may be a *quiet,* congested sounding cough, but in many cases there is no cough at all. Management consists of antibiotics and supportive care.

How does a doctor diagnose viral as opposed to bacterial pneumonia?

It is usually not difficult to differentiate viral from bacterial pneumonias since viral pneumonia is so much more common. Blood counts and chest x-rays can sometimes be helpful. The pediatrician considers many things before deciding whether to prescribe antibiotics. Bacterial pneumonias resolve quickly with antibiotics and of course viral pneumonias are unaffected.

My son has had a loud, very deep cough for 2 weeks. How can I tell if it is pneumonia?

"Deep" loud coughs are not characteristic of pneumonia but are an effort to clear mucus from the back of the throat. If your son had viral pneumonia, he would be recovering by this time; if he had bacterial pneumonia, you would have sought medical care long before now.

My daughter has had a bad cold for the past week. Instead of getting better, she's gotten worse in the last day or so. Her fever has come back and she just lays on the couch all day. Could she have pneumonia?

Possibly. Although cold symptoms can linger unchanged for many days before improving, a *deterioration* in your child's overall condition can signal a secondary bacterial infection such as pneumonia or sinusitis.

My son has had a bad cold with fever and wheezing for the past week. He coughs all day and night and isn't getting any better. Could he have pneumonia?

Possibly. If your son is not asthmatic and does not have a history of wheezing, it is likely that he has viral pneumonia.

Cough*

Cough is a protective reflex to clear the airways of irritating agents. Coughs in children are usually signs of colds, allergies, or asthma. Cough can sometimes be associated with viral or bacterial pneumonia, especially when there are no other upper respiratory tract symptoms. Coughing frequently bothers the parents more than the child. If a child is otherwise well and does not seem bothered by his coughing, it is okay to just leave him alone. If the child is ill or if the cough is interfering with the child's or parents' activities (including sleeping), he should be examined by the pediatrician.

Coughing in itself is not generally a reliable indicator of the seriousness of the child's condition. Fever, appetite, energy level, wheezing, and upper respiratory symptoms are much more important in deciding if the cough is a sign of more serious illness.

When should I worry about my child's cough?

Coughing that is continuous throughout the day and night without intervening quiet periods is of greater concern than intermittent "throat-clearing" coughs. Coughs associated with allergies or wheezing may signal

---

*See also asthma, allergic rhinitis, colds, croup, and pneumonia.

asthma. Persistent coughs in children who also have fever or loss of appetite and energy are more worrisome than persistent coughs in children who are running around in the yard "coughing their heads off." Barely audible, "quiet" coughs are of greater concern than loud, deep coughs. Croupy, barking coughs can be scary but are usually not serious.

My child coughs so hard she vomits! What does that mean?

Vomiting after paroxysms of coughing is extremely common in children and is just another way of clearing mucus. The presence of vomiting does not mean the cough is more serious. (Incidentally, asthmatics were once given medicines to make them vomit.)

Isn't there any relief for bothersome coughs?

Treatment of coughing consists of treatment of the underlying cause if it is treatable. Since a cough frequently lingers long after the provoking agent has disappeared, a cough suppressant such as Benadryl at bedtime can be indicated in some circumstances.

Green, Runny Nose and Sinus Infections

Like coughing, a green, runny nose in and of itself is not a good indicator of the seriousness of a child's illness. By far the most common causes are colds and allergies, neither of which can be treated with antibiotics. As the cold resolves naturally and the allergens disappear from the environment, the green, runny discharge goes away. Antibiotics will not speed things along.

When should I worry?

When associated with other systemic symptoms such as fever, irritability, loss of appetite and energy, pain, facial or eye swelling, and chronic continuous cough, a *persistent* (longer than 7 to 10 days) green, runny nose can signal a sinus or ear infection. These children are really sick and can benefit from antibiotics.

How long should I let my child go before I get him checked by the doctor?

If your child does not have any other systemic symptoms except for a green, runny nose, he does not need to be seen by a doctor at all. If he has systemic symptoms that do not seem to be improving by the seventh to tenth day, he should be examined. A green, runny nose that has been present for less than a week will not clear up any faster with medication.

Should I let my daughter go to school with a green, runny nose?

She can go to school if she feels well enough to do so and does not have a fever.

Vomiting and Diarrhea

When they occur together, vomiting and diarrhea are symptoms of an insult to the gastrointestinal tract, usually from a virus, bacteria, poison, or contaminated food. They are usually short lived, and investigation of the cause is usually limited to an interview with the mom. Vomiting is the presenting symptom and generally lasts only a few hours and almost always is over in 24 hours. Diarrhea follows and can last from 1 to 10 days or so depending on the cause. The only danger from vomiting and diarrhea, no matter what the cause, is dehydration. Because of their size, younger, smaller children are more at risk of dehydration than older children.

How do I keep my baby from getting dehydrated?

Because gastrointestinal illness is usually short lived, there is little risk of significant dehydration in a child who continues to take fluids throughout the illness. Offer breast milk or formula frequently. Avoid changing formula. If she won't take breast milk or formula, even the smallest, sickest babies can remain hydrated with teaspoonsful of rehydrating fluid such as Pedialyte offered every 10 or 15 minutes.

How do I know if my baby is getting enough fluid?

If she is alert and active and continues to take fluids, she's doing okay no matter how many times she's vomited or how many diapers she has dirtied. If she is listless, has a dry mouth and tongue, and is not urinating as often, she needs to be seen by the doctor.

Do I need to put my toddler on a bland or BRAT* diet?

No. Older children can drink water, sports drinks, and soft drinks and eat anything they want until the illness runs its course.

Anything? He would just eat cookies, french fries, and ice cream. Is that okay?

Most kids really don't want anything, but if they do, it's a good sign that they are getting well. This is not a good time to encourage a well-balanced diet.

---

*Bananas, rice, applesauce, and toast.

What about milk and juice?

Milk is okay, but most kids lose their appetite for it when they are sick. The high sugar content of fruit juice aggravates diarrhea and is not recommended.

What do I do if he won't eat anything at all?

He knows what he's doing. Keep offering fluids and things that you know he ordinarily loves and he'll eat when he's ready. A regular diet should be resumed as soon as possible during a gastrointestinal illness. Children will catch up fast once they feel better. Don't worry about it.

Don't I need to give him something for his vomiting and diarrhea?

Vomiting resolves quickly and does not require treatment. Diarrheas caused by an identifiable bacteria can sometimes be treated, but it's usually not necessary. (Frequently the child is well before the lab report gets back to the doctor.) Persistent diarrhea in a child who is otherwise well can sometimes be treated with Imodium.

Sore Throat, Strep Throat, and Rheumatic Fever, Scarlet Fever, Tonsillitis/Pharyngitis, and Mononucleosis

Tonsils are the infection-fighting glands of the throat. They are the "gate-keepers," and in the presence of invading microbes they can swell and bring blood and infection-fighting white cells ("pus") to the area to prevent further entry into the body. The tonsils are good at what they do. That's why tonsillitis is common and pneumonia isn't. Not much gets past the tonsils, but sometimes they take a pretty bad hit.

As with most pediatric illnesses, sore throats are most commonly caused by viruses. Depending on the age of the child and the time of year, strep throat represents up to 30% of sore throats.

What exactly is strep?

There are many kinds of streptococcal bacteria, but only group A beta-hemolytic strep (GABHS) is of any significance in the throat. Since there are many types of GABHS, you can get a strep throat many times. Other kinds of strep that cause pneumonia, sinusitis, ear and skin infections, etc. may or may not be GABHS.

What's the difference between sore throat, tonsillitis, and pharyngitis?

Tonsillitis refers to enlarged, red, painful tonsils with or without pus or ulcerations. Pharyngitis refers to infection in the rest of the throat and always involves some degree of tonsillitis whether obvious or not. Tonsillitis and pharyngitis go hand in hand and there's no need to differentiate between the two. It's all just a sore throat to me.

How can you tell if it's strep or not?

We can't know for sure unless a throat culture is done. Some signs and symptoms increase the probability that it's strep: headache, stomachache, tender glands in the neck, pus on the tonsils, fever, predisposition to strep, school age, and cold months. None of these is prerequisite to a diagnosis of a strep throat, but when some are present, it increases the likelihood that it's strep.

What are "swollen glands" anyway?

These are additional areas of specialized infection-fighting tissue that are interspersed throughout the body but are concentrated in areas around the main trunk of the body (i.e., the neck, armpits, and groin). Tonsils and adenoids are just glands that have special names. If a germ gets past the tonsils, another set of glands a little farther down the chain is called into play. Strep does this more often and that is why it is frequently associated with swollen glands, but many viruses can also do this.

My daughter hates to go to the doctor because she is so afraid of the tongue depressor. Can't you just use your judgment?

A physician can never be sure if a throat infection is caused by strep or not just by looking and asking questions. It can look and act like strep and not be strep; it can look and act like a virus and sometimes still be strep.

Why would the doctor do a throat culture if she doesn't even complain of a sore throat?

Frequently school-age children with strep throat will not complain of a sore throat at all but rather of a stomachache or a headache. Younger children may just vomit.

Does she have to have a culture every time she gets a sore throat, stomachache, or headache?

No. When symptoms are clearly due to a cold or other easily recognized virus or chronic drip from allergy, a culture is not necessary. When they are not, strep is frequently the culprit and a culture is warranted.

What's the difference between a culture and those 10-minute tests?

A culture is more accurate in identifying strep, but it takes 2 days to get the final result. The rapid 10-minute tests are very good (around 90% accuracy), but that's not considered good enough since a culture is cheap, easy to do, and is more accurate. When positive, a rapid test is enough to justify starting treatment, but when negative, a follow-up culture is needed to "double check" before deciding to withhold antibiotic treatment.

Sometimes my doctor doesn't do a test but just goes ahead and treats for strep. Is that okay?

Occasionally a physician may forego a culture and decide to treat for strep based on the presence of all the classic signs. It is unwise, however, to skip the culture just because the classic signs are not present; it can still be strep.

Sometimes the rapid test is negative and he treats her anyway. What's the point?

A doctor should always rely on his experience and clinical judgment since no test is perfect (inadequate specimen, faulty processing of the swab, poorly performed test, or inaccurate reporting of the result). If the follow-up culture is also negative, that confirms treatment can be stopped.

Wouldn't it be better to go ahead and start treatment and then just stop the antibiotics if the culture is negative?

Sounds good but it's not that simple. There are pros and cons to starting antibiotics before the culture result is known and to delaying antibiotics for 2 days pending the culture result.

Early treatment makes the child feel better sooner, shortens the contagious period, and gets everyone back on schedule sooner. Early treatment has the disadvantages of subjecting patients to unnecessary treatment since most sore throats are *not* caused by strep. In addition, there is some evidence that early treatment may result in more recurrences of strep throat a few weeks later.

Delayed treatment has the advantages of avoiding unnecessary antibiotics when a sore throat turns out not to be strep and allows the child to develop some immunity when it is. Delayed treatment has the disadvantages of postponing the relief of symptoms and increasing the time of contagiousness.

**Rapid tests, throat cultures, early treatment, delayed treatment—
no wonder I'm so confused and seem to get so many different opinions.
What's the best thing to do?**

Each individual case is different. Talk the options over with your doctor. I generally try to get patients to delay treatment until the culture results are known. I'd rather preschoolers "be sick" for a couple of days while awaiting final culture results because they are less likely to have strep, have no pressing commitments, and they benefit by building up immunities early. I generally end up treating older children who feel bad and have to get back to school. I try to get parents to wait for culture results if it is over the weekend and in summer months. Many other variables have to be considered, but this is a good starting place.

What will happen to my child if she has strep and isn't treated appropriately?

The sore throat will resolve on its own in 3 to 4 days. However, the reason it is important to treat strep throat is not to make the throat feel better sooner but to prevent an unusual but serious complication known as rheumatic fever.

What is rheumatic fever?

It is an immunologically mediated complication of strep throat. The heart is attacked by infection-fighting cells and is damaged.

Does delayed therapy increase the risk for rheumatic fever?

No. Antibiotics can be delayed 10 days and probably even longer without increasing the risk for rheumatic fever.

What's the best antibiotic for strep throat?

GABHS is still universally susceptible to penicillin and it is the drug of choice in nonallergic individuals; erythromycin is the drug of choice for penicillin-allergic individuals.

Why does my doctor use amoxicillin?

Amoxicillin is a penicillin derivative that tastes a little better and can be given less often. However, now that it is believed that one or two daily doses of penicillin are sufficient, this is no longer a good reason to use amoxicillin.

What about a penicillin shot?

Antibiotic injections do not work any faster or better than oral antibiotics, but they can be used in children who are vomiting if early treatment is indicated.

Is there a "stronger" antibiotic than penicillin?

The newer, "stronger" antibiotics may kill many other germs in addition to strep, but they are not better at killing strep than penicillin.

How long and how often is the medicine taken?

A full 10 days. In the past attempts to shorten the course of penicillin therapy have resulted in an increase in the incidence of rheumatic fever. However, twice-daily and probably even once-daily therapy is adequate, not three or four times a day as prescribed in the past.

Several shorter regimens that use some of the new "longer acting" antibiotics are being tested as treatment for strep throat. Most effectively eradicate the strep, but it is still uncertain if this will result in an increase in the incidence of rheumatic fever. If history is worth anything, caution is advised.

Is another culture necessary at the end of therapy to make sure it is gone?

No. If a child is well, it is not necessary to reculture at the end of the 10 days. Positive cultures at the end of therapy do not increase the risk of rheumatic fever. If children are no longer sick, additional therapy has no benefit.

When one of my children tests positive for strep throat, shouldn't the others be tested also?

No. Siblings and other close contacts of children with strep should not be "checked out" unless they show some signs of illness.

Why not prevent it or "nip it in the bud"?

Strep can be found in the throats of people who are not ill (so-called carriers). Their cultures will be positive, and they will unnecessarily be given 10 days of penicillin therapy. Within a couple of days after completing therapy the bacteria can reappear. Penicillin therapy is not used to prevent a carrier from becoming sick because it only works while taking the penicillin. Theoretically, that person would have to take it forever.

Isn't there any treatment for carriers?

Some antibiotics can eradicate the carrier state for a while (weeks perhaps). These can be used when a family keeps passing strep around to each other, necessitating an endless round of antibiotics.

Can carriers get rheumatic fever?

An asymptomatic person who has strep germs in the throat is not at risk for rheumatic fever. However, carriers can occasionally succumb to strep and become sick. If untreated, there is a theoretical risk of rheumatic fever, but some experts believe that the risk is actually lower in carriers. All patients who are symptomatic need 10 full days of therapy.

Are carriers contagious to others?

Theoretically, yes, but in real life probably not very. In the cold winter months up to 35% of people are walking around with strep germs in their throats and feel fine. If strep throats were that readily passed on to others, there would be a much higher incidence of strep throat and rheumatic fever.

Penicillin often doesn't work for my daughter's strep throats. How can this be if these organisms are susceptible to penicillin?

It probably wasn't strep that made her sick. She may be a carrier and her sore throats were in fact caused by viruses. A strep carrier is just as susceptible to other viral throat infections as anyone else. When cultured, she will be positive for strep even though her illness is viral. Since you can never be sure, she will have to be treated for 10 days.

I warn that the penicillin I prescribe for sore throat may not work because it looks like a viral infection to me even though the rapid test or culture was positive for strep. If viral in origin, they will not get well overnight as would be expected for a strep infection. It spares me a lot of irate phone calls.

My daughter has a lot of sore throats and many of these are strep. Amoxicillin doesn't seem to be working anymore. Shouldn't we try something stronger?

There are many types of GABHS, and it is just bad luck that she keeps getting reinfected. GABHS is still universally susceptible to penicillin and nothing will work better. If she is not responding, it is probably because some of her sore throats are caused by viruses. The next time her culture is positive for strep, try to hold off a few days before starting treatment and let her build up some immunity to the strep.

What about taking out her tonsils?

Removing the tonsils does not cut down on the number of infections. There is plenty of other tissue in the throat that can become infected and cause pain and illness.

I know some kids that have had their tonsils out and their moms say that they are doing so much better. Why?

Tonsils are removed when they get so big that they chronically obstruct the airway and cause symptoms such as snoring and poor growth. Tonsils shrink with time, and patients suffer fewer infections as they get older. It's unusual to have to remove tonsils. However, when large, obstructing tonsils are removed, patients greatly improve in many ways, but decreasing the number of infections is not necessarily one of them.

The last time she had strep throat it turned into scarlet fever! What can I do to stop that from happening again?

Nothing. Strep throat does not "turn into" scarlet fever. Scarlet fever is strep throat accompanied by a rash. It is caused by a particular strain of strep that produces a substance that turns the skin red, but it is no more serious than any other strep infection. It acts like and is treated like any other strep throat. It is still treated with penicillin, but penicillin will not affect the natural course of the rash, which resolves on its own in a couple of days.

Enough about strep. Is there anything I should know about viral sore throats?

With the exception of infectious mononucleosis, viral sore throats run their course in a few days or less without treatment. Many of these are also associated with red rashes resembling scarlet fever or penicillin allergy, especially in infants. Motrin can be used to control pain if the child is taking fluids well, and gargling with warm water helps if the child will cooperate.

What is "mono"?

Infectious mononucleosis is caused by a virus known as Epstein-Barr (EB) virus belonging to the herpes family.

Is it caused by kissing?

Not necessarily. The EB virus is spread like other respiratory viruses, which is usually from the hands to mouths and noses. Kissing is not necessarily the cause, but the direct exchange of saliva is probably a pretty good way of passing it on.

Is it serious?

In young children mono can be asymptomatic or run a course much like that of a mild viral illness. In older children and especially teenagers the sore throat from mono is usually much more severe and patients are much sicker for longer (up to 6 weeks or so). They have additional symptoms, particularly loss of energy and appetite. They frequently get a red rash if given ampicillin (on the assumption that it is strep throat), and this can be confused with scarlet fever or ampicillin allergy.

Why is it so much worse in older kids?

Most older children and adults infected with EB virus are asymptomatic or have mild symptoms. The ones that get really sick mount an overly aggressive immunologic response to the virus or the virus overwhelms the defense mechanisms of the body.

How do you tell mono from other viral sore throats?

You can't be sure early in the course of the illness, and blood tests for mono are not positive until at least 7 to 10 days after the onset of symptoms. If a sore throat does not resolve by then and the patient is still ill, a test for mono should be done.

My son had mono. He's better now, but the doctor won't let him play sports for 6 weeks. Why not?

Mono affects the whole body, not just the throat. Liver involvement can result in mild to moderate hepatitis. Spleen involvement results in an enlarged, congested, friable spleen that can be easily damaged if traumatized. Until the liver and spleen return to normal, it is advisable to avoid potentially injurious activities.

Is there a treatment for mono?

Like most viral illnesses, the course of mono cannot be altered with medication. Steroid therapy can be tried cautiously in some adolescents who are particularly miserable or who are slow to recover since steroids blunt the inflammatory response and can lessen symptoms. Acyclovir is sometimes tried, but with questionable success.

Does mono lead to chronic fatigue syndrome?

This is a subject of much debate. I don't know. Herpesviruses such as the EB virus that causes mono are known to inhabit the body for life, so it's a distinct possibility. However, just like the herpes infections that cause recurrent shingles, genital herpes, and cold sores, other factors may be more important than the history of viral infection. If chronic fatigue syndrome turns out to be a late complication of EB viral infection, it is unlikely that antiviral medications will be any more successful than they are for other late herpesvirus complications.

Ear Infections

MIDDLE EAR INFECTIONS (OTITIS MEDIA)

Otitis media is the result of an obstructed eustachian tube (ET), which runs between the back of the nose and the middle ear. The function of this tube is to equalize the pressure between the air-filled middle ear space and the outside world. This is the source of "pops" when going up in a plane or down to the bottom of a pool. When the ET dysfunctions, fluid is drawn in to fill the middle ear space to equalize the pressure.

Why do little children get so many ear infections?

A better question would be, "Why do little children get so much ear pain and discomfort?" In children the ET is very small, and when it is swollen or plugged by mucus in the nose as a result of a cold or allergy, there is discomfort or pain. If it stays this way for 12 hours or so, fluid is drawn into the middle ear space to equalize the pressure. This usually resolves the acute pain, although the feeling of fullness in the ears may be uncomfortable at first.

How do you know if it's an obstruction or an infection?

If the obstruction continues without intermittent relief for several days, eventually a bacterial infection may ensue. Inflammation sets in, the pain returns, and the eardrum becomes red and bulges with pus.

What does it mean when my baby pulls and rubs her ears?

In most cases, nothing, especially when it is the only symptom. Once babies discover their ears they commonly calm themselves this way. Babies may grab at their ears when there is discomfort from teething, sore throats, or ear infection, but there will be other symptoms in addition to the ear pulling.

Why does the ear pain come and go? My son's up all night crying and complaining, but when I take him to the pediatrician the next morning, he says it doesn't even hurt! The doctor must think I'm crazy!

I hear this story many times every single day. Pain will come and go as the ET plugs and unplugs, just as a nose plugs and unplugs variably during the course of a cold. As the cold resolves over 7 to 10 days, so does the swelling and mucous production and the ET will remain open. The ear pain will then resolve once and for all.

Why does the pain always seem to be worse at night?

Pain is generally worse at night for many reasons, one of which is that there is less distraction from the pain when lying in bed in the dark. Another important reason relates to gravity. When a child is vertical during the day, gravity decreases swelling and facilitates drainage. When a child is horizontal, there is increased pressure on the eardrum. This is why he wants you to hold him upright and won't let you cradle his head down on your shoulder. It explains why you can quiet him, but he cries out again when you start to lay him down.

Why doesn't this happen to me when I have a cold or allergy?

Older children and adults have fewer ear problems because the ET is much larger and they can blow their noses and clear their throats. The ET is less likely to become plugged.

Won't antibiotics prevent all this or "nip it in the bud"?

Although antibiotic therapy has been the standard treatment for ear pain, it is obvious to anyone whose child has "ear infections" that it does not work well. It can still take 2 to 3 days to get relief, and by then the pain probably goes away because the ET opened up naturally.

Can't the infection spread if it isn't treated with antibiotics?

In Europe it is not routine practice to treat ear pain with antibiotics. They have no more complications than we do in the United States and much less problems with antibiotics. Europeans treat the pain as needed and let time take care of the obstruction, usually 2 to 3 days.

When do you prescribe antibiotics?

I reserve antibiotics for cases of true bacterial infection that occur after several days of unrelieved, persistent obstruction when symptoms should be resolving (at least 7 to 10 days).

What happens if antibiotics aren't started as soon as ear pain develops?

Studies are variable, but ear symptoms in approximately 85% of children who do not receive antibiotics will disappear within 2 to 3 days (about the same time it takes an antibiotic to "work"). Intermittent pain or discomfort may occur as the ET opens and closes, but this is not the result of bacteria and antibiotics will not alleviate this.

What about the other 15%?

Unfortunately, life is not fair; some children will have complications, in this case bacterial infection. For this group, antibiotics will work quickly and easily.

What predisposes some kids to bacterial infections and not others?

Some well-known risk factors for true bacterial infection are prematurity, young age, male gender, day care, history of allergies, siblings, smokers in the household, family history of ear problems, and cold weather months. All these risk factors are so common it is surprising that *only* 15% of kids develop actual bacterial infection.

My son has a green, runny nose and several risk factors for ear infection. What's wrong with starting treatment early just in case?

The casual and indiscriminate use of antibiotics for green, runny nose and ear pain has resulted in an "antibiotics arms race." For example, Katie has a bad cold and on day 3 her nasal discharge is green. She has a fever and last night complained of an earache. The pediatrician saw her the next morning and prescribed amoxicillin. Two days later Katie is still fussy, up at night, and pulling at her ears. Mom calls back to say that the amoxicillin isn't working and the pediatrician prescribes Ceclor.

Why didn't the amoxicillin work?

The amoxicillin didn't work because the pain was due to obstruction, not infection, and she also had a pretty miserable cold. The Ceclor *seemed* to work because by then the cold and obstruction were improving anyway.

Now, it's 2 weeks later and Katie has another cold. This time she's brought in "right away" to avoid that nasty ear infection again. Of course her ears are red (as are her throat, nose, and eyes; she has a cold!) and she's labeled "prone" to bad ear infections that require "strong" antibiotics. Katie is prescribed Ceclor at the start since it worked so well last time.

Well, this time the Ceclor doesn't work for the same reason the amoxicillin didn't work last time. Mom calls back a couple of days later and requests an even "stronger" antibiotic, let's say Biaxin. Lo and behold, the Biaxin works for the same reason the Ceclor worked last time, that is, ear pain usually resolves on its own in a day or two. Now, however, Katie has developed a reputation for "terrible ear infections."

Poor Katie. It's winter, she's in day care, and she gets another cold only 10 days later. Katie's resistance is wearing down now and the frequent viral insults are taking their toll. This time she gets a bona fide bacterial infection. She has persistent, unremitting pain and mom calls the doctor quickly. She has a rip-roaring, red eardrum that's bulging with pus. She vomits all over the doctor.

Since she's vomiting and can't keep oral antibiotics down, she gets a shot of Rocephin and is given a prescription for Biaxin since it's the only antibacterial that hasn't had a chance to fail yet. Three days later Katie still has a fever and is not improving because her cold has peaked. This time mom and the doctor decide to "give it a little more time" (translation: "there's nothing else I can do").

It's now 10 days and mom is upset and frustrated; she is worried about Katie's system being exposed to all these antibiotics. Katie is no better and now has diarrhea and a rash. This time she is really infected with bacteria. Katie is now on the "antibiotic not-so-merry-go-round." (Pharmaceutical stocks skyrocket again!) There's a good chance Katie will end up with tubes in her ears.

How could this have been avoided?

Had Katie's ear pain been treated with appropriate pain medication (codeine if necessary) for the 1 or 2 days that she needed it rather than with antibiotics, she would have felt much better, much sooner, almost immediately, in fact. The bacterial infection she experienced with cold No. 3 could not have been prevented in any case (her immune system was worn down), but amoxicillin would have treated the ear infection easily.

Isn't withholding antibiotic treatment risky?

Studies indicate that "untreated" ear pain is no more likely to result in serious complications later on than antibiotic-treated ear pain. In fact, when a complication does develop in an "untreated" child, it can be more easily treated with standard antibiotics. A complication in a "treated" child is likely to be the result of infection by bacteria that were resistant to the previously used antibiotics.

Won't it affect the child's hearing?

Anybody with fluid in their ear, whether infected or not, will not hear well until the fluid clears. This takes time and most pediatricians and ENTs don't start to worry about this temporary loss of hearing unless it persists for at least 3 months with no hope in sight for clearing or if the child's speech and language development is being affected.

I thought ear infections can cause deafness. Is that not true?

In the old days antibiotics were not used to treat ear pain and infections. Children endured the pain until it resolved on its own, occasionally by spontaneous rupture of the eardrum and subsequent drainage of the middle ear space. Those who were taken to the doctor often had their eardrum lanced for immediate pain relief and drainage. Where are all these deaf people?

How long does it take an ear infection to clear up?

Bacterial infection of the middle ear has a predictable course. If the bacteria are susceptible to the chosen antibiotic, the germs will be eliminated within 48 hours, probably sooner. The inflammatory reaction, the redness, pain, and swelling, may take another couple of days to subside. The fluid, however, may take a few days to several *months* to clear.

Why does it take so long for the fluid to clear up in some children?

No one knows why, but the body is known for its tendency to keep reacting to irritants even after they are gone. (Fluid-filled ears are more common in children with allergies.) Also children frequently get a series of colds, often intermixed with allergies, and the body never has time to completely "clean up" one insult before a new one comes along.

Would decongestants or antihistamines dry up the ear any faster?

No. Decongestants and antihistamines have never been successful in "drying up" the ears. Remember that decongestants and antihistamines have side effects that can actually increase the viscosity of mucous secretions, making them harder to clear, as well as interfere with the body's natural defenses in other ways. Together these factors may act to *encourage* bacterial infection.

I've heard that steroids might work. Is that the case?

There is some evidence that steroids may work by turning off the inflammatory response, but it's still controversial. Of course, there are significant side effects from steroid use that must be factored in.

If my child has an ear infection, can I take him on an airplane?

Children fly with real and imagined ear infections all the time. All young kids tend to cry and fuss on airplanes, so who's to know? There is more risk for ear pain in the first days of a cold when the ET isn't functioning well, but this happens on the ground as well as in the air. Staying home won't make any difference.

Does that mean yes or no?

It means yes. It's okay for kids to fly with ear infections. Scientifically speaking, once fluid has been drawn into the middle ear (which is the case with an ear infection), pressure equalization is achieved. Fluid-filled spaces are not affected by the pressure changes of altitude as are air-filled spaces, so there is actually *less* risk of experiencing ear pain with fluid-filled ears than with normal air-filled middle ear spaces. Well kids and everyone else on the airplane are at the mercy of the first officer's ability to keep the cabin pressure constant.

What if time and antibiotics don't clear up the fluid?

At one time painful ears were lanced on the spot (e.g., kitchen table). This immediately relieved the pain and drained the fluid and no further treatment was necessary. I'm certain that was quite a spectacle, and it must have been a welcome relief for everyone when antibiotics came along. Now that antibiotics are no longer the "wonder drugs" they once were, we have PE tubes and adenoidectomy.

What are adenoids and PE tubes?

Adenoids are the equivalent of tonsils that are found back behind the nose. They enlarge with infection or allergy and can obstruct the nasal passages and ET. PE (pressure equalization) tubes are tiny plastic tubes inserted into the eardrum to allow for equalization of pressure when the ET is not able to effectively do this, that is, they "lance" the eardrums. What goes around, comes around. PE tubes are inserted in a surgical suite.

Which children benefit from adenoidectomy and PE tubes?

PE tubes and adenoidectomy can be used to clear the fluid and to prevent future obstruction in children whose ears cause chronic problems, who can't hear well, and who are unlikely to get better anytime soon (those who are young, in day care, allergic, and during winter). PE tubes are placed to improve hearing, but they have the added advantage of preventing middle ear obstruction (especially when combined with adenoidectomy) and thus can cut down on the number of infections also.

What happens if ears get infected even with tubes in place?

When an infection occurs despite tubes, there is little or no pain because there is no buildup of pressure. In those who continue to react to irritants even after they are gone, the PE tubes can continue to drain fluid for weeks. Most pediatricians and ENTs will try a round or two of antibiotics, but if that was expected to work, the tubes wouldn't have been inserted in the first place.

My son has PE tubes. I've heard differing opinions on whether he needs ear plugs when he's in the bath or pool. What do you think?

This is the subject of much debate. Those who are pro plugs strongly feel that water is not good for the middle ear and should be kept out with custom-designed ear plugs or with cotton soaked in Vaseline and securely placed in the ear canals. Those against ear plugs acknowledge that water is not good for the middle ear but that it is impossible to keep out every single drop of water with plugs, especially in kids who fiddle with them. They believe that *trapped* drops of water are more harmful than water flowing freely in and out.

So what should I do?

You have two choices (1) Since it's a toss-up, take the easy way out—no plugs. If he keeps getting a lot of infections, hang your head low and start using plugs. (2) Since it's a toss-up, try to keep all the water out—use plugs. If he keeps getting a lot of infections, hang your head low and stop using plugs.

Do the PE tubes and adenoidectomy justify the risk of anesthesia and surgery?

Adenoidectomy and PE tubes are usually a significant improvement over the antibiotic not-so-merry-go-round because it immediately improves hearing and relieves pain.

What can I do to avoid this mess in the first place?

It's best to avoid the whole scenario by not using antibiotics for ear pain in the first place. Save them for legitimate bacterial infections. I also advise against the routine use of decongestants and antihistamines for the treatment of cold symptoms.

The heyday of casual, inappropriate antibiotic use is over, but 25 years of prescribing practices aren't going to change overnight. Many physicians just keep doing what they've always done and then refer the child to someone else if it doesn't work. The message is getting out, but not fast enough for all those kids with tubes in their ears (including two of my own three) or kids with cancer who die of untreatable infection.

SWIMMER'S EAR (EXTERNAL OTITIS)

External otitis is a very different illness than otitis media. It is an infection of the skin of the ear canal. It is easily differentiated from otitis media by severe, unremitting pain when the ear (especially the little triangle at the front of the ear) is touched or bumped. It is not associated with any other upper respiratory symptoms such as congestion, fever, or cough. Swimmer's ear occurs in children older than those who get otitis media since they are the ones who spend a lot of time underwater.

Can middle ear infection and swimmer's ear occur at the same time?

I never say never, but it is extremely unlikely.

I'm real good about cleaning the wax out my child's ears, but he still gets infections. What can I do?

Wax is not dirt. It is the ears' protective coating. It is meant to keep irritants such as wind and water and germs out of the ear and off the delicate skin of the ear canal. When wax is removed by scrubbing or washed out over time with pool, sea, or lake water, the ear is no longer protected and is ripe for irritation and then infection.

My son loves the water. What can I do to keep him from getting swimmer's ear?

Swimmer's ear is easy to prevent by decreasing trauma to the ear canal (lay off the Q-tips) and by drying the ear (towel or blow dryer) after prolonged periods of swimming. Kids who are in the water a lot will lose the protective wax over time, so it's a good idea to try to dry the ear as best as you can and instill a solution of 50% alcohol/50% vinegar into the ears after a long day of swimming to kill any lingering germs.

I've been doing this after he gets out of the pool, but he's starting to complain of some tenderness. What now?

Even if an infection occurs, the alcohol/vinegar antibiotic solution used four to six times daily can usually abort it. If it doesn't improve within a day or two, you'll need to try something else.

Once the infection has progressed, the ear canal can become so swollen that medication cannot get in. The doctor can then prescribe a combination steroid/antibiotic suspension.

Why don't we just use that in the first place?

You can, but you probably already have rubbing alcohol and white vinegar in the house. The alcohol/vinegar solution is as good at killing the germs as traditional antibiotics. The commonly prescribed antibiotic eardrops have a steroid in them to decrease the inflammatory response (swelling) and make it easier for the antibiotic to get down into the ear, but early in an infection there isn't much swelling and the steroid isn't needed.

My doctor prescribed *eye*drops?

There are similar preparations for treating eye infections that have the same active ingredients but are more "gentle" and less likely to burn an irritated ear. I use them too.

Can you give me some of those eardrops for pain?

Sure, but they don't work that well. Swimmer's ear can be extremely painful, and I would also use Motrin. In the worst cases an ear wick and codeine may be needed.

What's an ear wick?

It is a sliver of cotton that is placed in the ear canal and then wetted with antibiotic/steroid solution. It expands to open a swollen ear canal and forces the medication into close contact with the irritated skin. It helps relieve the pain much like wrapping a swollen ankle does. Generally infections this severe will also require an oral antibiotic.

How long must my son stay out of the water?

It is best to stay out of the water until the symptoms are clearly subsiding and this takes at least 3 days or so. Discourage him from going underwater for as many days as you can and dry the ears and put in his medicine when he gets out.

Pinkeye

"Pinkeye" is the term commonly used to describe the condition in which the whites of the eyes, the conjunctivae, turn red. It is also used to describe matting of the eyelashes and drainage in the corners of the eyes from swollen, pink eyelids, even though the conjunctiva is white. These two conditions are more correctly termed "conjunctivitis" and "blepharitis," respectively.

BLEPHARITIS

Does it really matter what you *call* it?

Not really, except that blepharitis can usually be managed at home by wiping out the eyes frequently with a warm, wet, clean cloth and keeping the hands and face clean. A little baby shampoo applied to the eyelashes can help. However, for most families, this is too much trouble and it's easier to just prescribe antibiotic eyedrops.

My child frequently has what you call blepharitis. There's green stuff in the corner of his eyes, but the whites aren't red. He's not sick at all, but the school sends him home anyway, saying it's pinkeye. He can't go back without a doctor's prescription for eyedrops or a note. What should I do?

This happens frequently. Blepharitis is much more common than conjunctivitis, but most everyone lumps the two conditions together and calls it pinkeye. Blepharitis is about as contagious as a sinus infection (not very contagious at all). He shouldn't be sent home from school for that unless he feels bad or has other associated symptoms.

How do I know if he needs antibiotic eyedrops or not?

If you are keeping his eyes, face, and hands clean and the "goop" in his eyes keeps reaccumulating (not just in the morning or after a nap), he'll probably need antibiotic drops.

Can I show this to our school nurse?

Sure. I hope you have better luck than I did with mine.

CONJUNCTIVITIS

When the whites of the eyes are red, it's conjunctivitis. There may or may not be drainage in the corners of the eyes or matting of the eyelashes and swollen, pink eyelids. The causes of conjunctivitis are viral, bacterial, and allergic.

Viral Conjunctivitis

Approximately 80% of the cases of conjunctivitis in children are due to viral causes ("a cold in the eye") and frequently are associated with a runny nose and other cold symptoms. There may or may not be a fever. Frequently the virus is limited to the conjunctiva and there are no associated symptoms except red, itchy, tearing eyes occasionally described as "sand in the eyes." Viral infections run their course in a few days without treatment, but some viruses can linger for up to 2 weeks. They are very contagious. Frequent eyewashes with sterile saline solution may make the child more comfortable if he will allow it.

If it's viral, why does my doctor always prescribe antibiotic eyedrops?

Although most conjunctivitis in children is viral in origin, frequent eye rubbing inevitably leads to a secondary bacterial infection. These kids have itchy eyes, dirty hands and nails, and runny noses. It only takes a couple of days or so for bacterial infection to set in. For this reason, I almost always prescribe antibiotic eyedrops for pinkeye with the warning that the drops may not seem to help at first.

My child hates to have drops placed in his eye four times a day. If it isn't going to help, anyway, do I have to do it?

No. It is also reasonable to try to avoid secondary bacterial infection and antibiotic drops by keeping the hands clean and off the face and washing the eyes out frequently with sterile saline solution. This is likely to work in older cooperative kids but is almost impossible in young kids.

Bacterial Conjunctivitis

Bacterial conjunctivitis is less common overall but is probably a more frequent cause of conjunctivitis in young children (younger than 3 years).

How can you tell bacterial from viral conjunctivitis?

Conjunctivitis caused by bacteria is usually not associated with other cold symptoms and seems to come on more suddenly. It is more likely to be associated with green or yellow drainage, eyelash matting, and mucus in the corners of the eyes that persist throughout the day, not just when the child wakes up in the morning. The whites of the eyes are red. Sometimes it is hard to decide if the conjunctivitis is viral or bacterial, but in younger children, even if it is viral to begin with, bacteria soon follow. Almost all kids will need to be treated with antibiotics.

My child woke up this morning with a red, puffy swollen eyelid. Should I worry?

Young children will sometimes have red, swollen, matted eyes that involve the *skin* of the eyelids and may even extend onto the skin of the face. The conjunctivae are not usually red. They become sick fairly rapidly. This is a cellulitis, an infection of the skin that surrounds the eyes, and is much more serious. The child needs a careful examination and systemic antibiotics.

Allergic Conjunctivitis

Allergic conjunctivitis looks like viral conjunctivitis just like an allergy can look like a cold. Older children can usually tell if their red, itchy eyes "feel like their allergies" or if they feel like they have a cold. Treatment for both consists of keeping the hands clean and away from the face and washing the eyes out as frequently as tolerated with sterile saline solution. If the child has a history of allergy, an anti-inflammatory eyedrop (not a steroid) or a topical or systemic antihistamine can be used. These children are still susceptible to secondary bacterial infection, and an antibiotic may need to be added in a few days if there is no improvement or the condition suddenly worsens.

My daughter started eyedrops for her pinkeye yesterday. Can she go back to school today?

It is hard to know what the cause of her "pinkeye" is, but chances are it is viral and it just has to run its course. The antibiotic drops are most likely for preventing or treating secondary bacterial infection. She can go back to school when her eyes are no longer red. If you are certain that her red eyes are just an allergic reaction, she should be able to go back if she shows no signs of bacterial infection, but good luck convincing the school of that!

Chickenpox and Shingles and Other Herpesvirus Infections

CHICKENPOX AND SHINGLES

Chickenpox (varicella) and shingles (zoster) are caused by the same varicella-zoster (VZ) virus, a member of the herpesvirus family. The initial infection with the VZ virus results in clinical chickenpox, which runs its course in about 7 to 10 days. As is the case with other herpesviruses, the VZ virus is not eradicated from the body but will continue to dwell in the nervous system for a person's lifetime. During periods of relative immunosuppression (old age, pregnancy, cancer, and stress) the virus can re-emerge and cause painful localized blisters known as shingles. About 95% of the population becomes infected with the VZ virus and has chickenpox in childhood. Those who don't get chickenpox until adolescence or adulthood have much more severe cases.

Isn't there a treatment for chickenpox now?

Acyclovir can decrease the symptoms when begun in the first 24 hours of the onset of the rash. Unless you are anticipating chickenpox because of a definite history of exposure, it is almost always too late to benefit from acyclovir once the diagnosis is made.

How long after an exposure will a susceptible child break out with chickenpox?

Since a child with chickenpox is contagious for up to 4 days *before* the appearance of the first lesion, it is often impossible to know when exposure occurred. The rash can appear from as early as the tenth day to as late as the twenty-first day after exposure.

How contagious is chickenpox?

Very. The attack rate in a family is approximately 80%. Chickenpox virus travels through air-conditioning and heating ducts and can infect susceptible individuals down the hall or on another floor.

What about the new vaccine?

Varivax is recommended for anyone over the age of 12 years who has not had chickenpox and for anyone over the age of 1 year who wants to avoid chickenpox.

Can you get chickenpox more than once?

It is unusual to get chickenpox again, but it can happen, especially in children who had a very mild case or have it before the age of 1 year.

Is is possible to have had chickenpox and not know it? My mom can't remember for sure.

Many adults who think that they never had chickenpox probably did have a mild case (one or two spots that looked like insect bites).

Would it hurt to get vaccinated if I had a mild case of chickenpox that went unrecognized?

No. As long as you are sure you are not pregnant and will not become pregnant for a couple of months it's okay to get the vaccine even if you aren't absolutely sure if you've had chickenpox.

Is there anyway to tell if I've had chickenpox or not?

A blood test is available to check for chickenpox immunity and can then be followed by vaccination if needed. This is important for women of childbearing age, especially if they have susceptible children who can infect them.

If I get chickenpox during pregnancy, can it hurt my baby?

Chickenpox infection in a mother can result in problems for her fetus.

What if I've already had chickenpox but my toddler comes down with it? Can this affect my unborn baby?

No. A fetus is not at risk if its mother is immune to chickenpox even if there is chickenpox in the household.

I just had a baby and my older daughter is at home with chickenpox. Can my newborn go home with me tomorrow?

No. A newborn baby is at serious risk if infected and cannot go home if a patient with chickenpox is present.

My daughter was diagnosed with shingles. She hasn't been around anyone with chickenpox. Where did she get it?

Shingles is not the result of exposure to someone with chickenpox. Shingles occurs when the original VZ virus re-emerges from its dormant state in the nervous system at times of decreased immunity.

Is she contagious?

When a person has shingles, active viruses are present in the lesions; that person is contagious to anyone who has not already had chickenpox.

It is really painful. Is there any treatment?

Shingles resolves on its own, but acyclovir may speed healing if started very early in the illness when the skin is sensitive or burns but the rash has not appeared. Steroids are used in some circumstances. Motrin is a good choice for pain control.

Can she get them again?

Shingles can recur throughout life, but it is unusual for healthy people to have more than one outbreak.

Is a fetus or newborn at risk if the mother gets shingles?

Shingles is not the original infection with the VZ virus and a mother has enough immunity to prevent any complications in her fetus. A newborn, however, is at risk from anyone who has shingles.

OTHER HERPESVIRUS INFECTIONS

There are many other viruses in the herpes family that can cause illness. Herpes simplex types 1 and 2 are responsible for cold sores and genital sores, respectively. Like other herpesvirus infections, the initial outbreak and illness are usually more severe. Recurrences become less frequent and less severe as the years go by. Recurrent lesions are the result of re-emergence of the virus, not new exposure to others, but recurrent lesions are contagious to others who have not been infected before.

My baby had a fever and some gum ulcers. My doctor said it was herpes! How could he get that?

The initial infection of herpes simplex type 1 occurs in the first 5 years or so of life in about 95% of the population. It is a routine childhood illness. It can go unnoticed (just "teething" or "fussy") or develop into serious illness with high fever, swollen, red gums, and many painful ulcers on the cheeks, gums, and tongue. It can last up to 14 days and is called herpetic gingivostomatitis. Kids can be so sick and in such pain that they require hospitalization for IV fluids and pain medication.

The doctor said my baby could get cold sores when he's older?

Cold sores on the outer surface of the lips are the result of re-emergence of this infection at times of relative immunosuppression.

My husband gets a lot of cold sores. Is this tendency inherited?

Yes. There is a genetic predisposition for cold sores. Your baby's herpetic gingivostomatitis may be a result of an inherited inability to fight herpes infection.

Are fever blisters *inside* the mouth caused by herpesvirus?

No. The presence of recurrent fever blisters inside the lips and on the gums and cheeks is known as aphthous stomatitis. It is not caused by herpesvirus and is not contagious. The cause of aphthous stomatitis is unknown, but it has a strong hereditary component.

I occasionally see teachers and children at preschool and school with cold sores on their lips. Are they contagious?

Anyone with a cold sore is contagious and should not be allowed around infants, who are at risk of developing serious problems. Toddlers and school-age children who have not been infected previously are also at risk, but they do not have serious problems and are bound to get cold sores sooner or later. Close contact is required for spread of infection, and this is more likely in a preschool than in a school setting. If it is school policy to permit children with lesions to attend, it should be required that the lesions be covered with antiviral ointment (acyclovir) to minimize the risk of spread.

Is there any treatment?

Acyclovir (topical or oral) has not been shown to alter the course significantly, but it may lessen the contagiousness to others.

What is roseola?

It is an infection with a herpesvirus known as HHV-6. Herpesviruses are responsible for roseola and several other viral illnesses in infants associated with high fever, rash, seizures, and meningitis.

I had no idea that herpesviruses were so common. Don't they cause serious infections?

These viruses are extremely common and severe illness is extremely rare. Presumably most infections are so mild they go unnoticed. Many episodes of "teething," "viral syndromes," "allergic reactions," and "febrile seizures" may actually be a herpesvirus infection of some sort.

I am pregnant and have a history of *recurrent* genital herpes. My doctor says I will have to have a cesarean section. Is that absolutely necessary?

No. Mothers who have a history of recurrent genital herpes lesions pose little or no risk to their fetus. However, many physicians still deliver these babies by cesarean section if there are active lesions present. In most cases this is probably not necessary.

I'm pregnant and just became infected with genital herpes. What should I do?

Primary infection with genital herpes during pregnancy is a serious concern near the time of delivery. Talk to your doctor. Cesarean section and acyclovir play important roles in treating primary genital herpes in mothers and newborns.

Are there any other herpesviruses I need to know about?

Infectious mononucleosis is caused by EB virus, which is another member of the herpesvirus family. It is generally a mild illness in young children (usually just another sore throat), but it can be debilitating in adolescents and adults.

Is it possible that chronic fatigue syndrome is caused by a herpesvirus?

Because of the tendency of herpesviruses to linger for life and re-emerge at will, the EB virus has been blamed for chronic fatigue syndrome. It is still controversial.

Since it's a herpesvirus, won't acyclovir help?

Acyclovir is an antiviral drug used to treat herpesviruses, but like all antiviral medications, it must be started very early in the illness and even then will only lessen the impact of the illness. By the time mono, chronic fatigue syndrome, or most other herpesvirus infections are diagnosed, it's too late to benefit from the modest effects of acyclovir.

What about steroids?

Steroids are tried for most frustrating, lingering problems. Occasionally they help, but there are so many side effects and concerns about steroids that routine use is not recommended.

Urinary Tract Infection, Genitourinary Itching, Pinworms, and Frequent Urination

Sooner or later little girls will complain of frequent urination, burning urination, or itchy "privates." Although it can happen to boys and girls, it seems that it's mostly a problem of 3- or 4-year-old girls. Mom is always concerned that her daughter has a bladder infection like she herself has had, but unless there's a previous history of urinary tract problems or unexplained fevers, this is unlikely.

What causes urinary tract infections?

First of all, we have to differentiate the two major kinds of urinary tract infections (UTI): upper tract or kidney infection and lower tract or bladder infection. Most people think of bladder infection when they think of UTI. These are caused by bacteria from the rectum ascending up the short urethras of little girls into the bladder and causing infection. This results in the typical burning pain and frequency of urination.

A kidney infection can be the result of ascending bacteria in some cases but can also be the result of a "blood infection" settling into the kidneys. It's a completely different disease process. When the kidney is involved, children are usually much sicker and may not even have the typical bladder symptoms of urinary frequency, burning, or itching.

Just because she's never had a UTI before, how can you be so sure it's not one this time?

The only way to be sure is to collect a midstream, clean catch urine specimen for urinalysis. Most physicians can do this in their office and rule out UTI right away. They can also send the urine to the lab to culture for bacteria to be absolutely certain. This takes a couple of days.

What's a midstream, clean catch urine specimen?

It is the best way to collect the urine without using a needle or a catheter. If the urine is not collected properly, you might as well not collect it at all. A poorly collected urine sample can contain skin cells, bacteria, and white and red blood cells that have been washed into it from the "contaminated" skin around the genital and anal areas and mistakenly lead to the diagnosis of UTI. It causes a big problem (more on that later).

Why don't they tell me how to do it right? The nurse usually just hands me a cup and some wipes.

I know. I usually try to explain the proper technique first, but sometimes urine collection cups are handed out indiscriminately at the reception desk for all urinary complaints and I don't get the chance.

How do I do it properly?

You and your daughter should both thoroughly wash your hands. Open three or four packages of the wipes, but remove them from the package one at a time as you need them. Carefully spread your little girl's legs open and wipe *once* from front to back and throw the wipe away. Do this several more times, wiping front to back only once with each wipe. Don't scrub. Take the lid off the cup. Then have your little girl sit on the toilet and spread her legs as wide as she comfortably can. Encourage her to urinate normally into the toilet. Once she has started to urinate, carefully move the collection cup into position to catch some of the urine stream. Collect only a little bit (half an inch is plenty) and then remove the cup. If you didn't get some of her urine on your hands, you probably didn't do it right. Put the lid on the cup and give it to the nurse.

What if it is a UTI?

A UTI in a child (girl or boy) is more significant than in an adult. One in three children with a confirmed UTI will have a congenital (present from birth) abnormality of the urinary tract that predisposed the child to infection. (This is why it is unusual for a child to have the first UTI after 3 years of age.) Almost every child with a confirmed UTI will need to have some kind of "imaging" studies (sonogram or special x-rays or nuclear scan) to make sure that no congenital or acquired urinary tract abnormality led to the infection. This is why it is so important not to send poorly collected specimens to the lab. If the sample shows evidence of infection, the child is subjected to a lot of unnecessary tests. *Please* tell the doctor if you had trouble collecting the specimen and save everyone a lot of grief.

How do you treat UTI?

The bacteria that cause UTI are easily treated with antibiotics. In "uncomplicated" cases only a day or two (perhaps only a single dose) of antibiotics may be needed, but physicians still traditionally prescribe a 10-day course. The pediatrician is more concerned about the possibility that some underlying urinary tract abnormality is responsible than about the presence of bacteria. Complicated cases of UTI require longer therapy.

What makes a UTI "complicated"?

We call it "complicated" if it involves the kidney, is recurrent, is caused by an underlying urinary tract abnormality, or is resistant to conventional antibiotics.

What if the urinary system is abnormal?

There are many abnormalities and so it depends on the type. Some abnormalities are outgrown, some can be treated with medication, and some require surgical intervention.

My daughter occasionally complains of itching and burning of the genitourinary region. The doctor always says her urine is "clear." What else can it be?

Itchy "privates" and burning on urination are most commonly caused by overaggressive hygiene and irritating commercial products, not UTI. Once irritated, little girls will scratch with their dirty hands and nails and cause even more irritation. Mom then steps up the hygiene and aggravates the problem even more.

How should I keep her clean?

A little girl's genital area is sufficiently cleansed by her own natural secretions and warm water. There is no need for scrubbing or soap. Sitting in a warm tub or showering is adequate.

Aren't baby bubble baths and shampoos gentle enough?

For most kids, yes, but if your daughter has had some problems, no. Bubble baths and shampoos can be very irritating to the genital area, even the ones advertised as "clinically mild." If your daughter has complained of itching or burning when she urinates, she should not use bubble bath or sit in the tub after her hair has been shampooed.

What can I do to make her feel better?

Once the problem is understood, it is easy to treat and results are usually seen in several days. Until the itching and burning subside, Vaseline mixed with a small dab of 1% hydrocortisone cream can be placed on the irritated area, and your little girl can be encouraged to urinate in the bathtub until the burning goes away. Keep her hands clean and her nails short.

The doctor says it's not a UTI and I've stopped all the bubble bath and shampoo. She's still itching and burning. Now what?

When this does not solve the problem, if it returns despite good hygienic practices, or if there is associated anal itching, there's a good chance that pinworms are contributing to the problem.

Pinworms! Where did she get *those?*

Pinworms are ubiquitous and are commonly present in the intestinal tract of humans. They usually cause no symptoms. They are passed hand to mouth, especially between kids whose toilet hygiene is less than optimal. Parents pick them up when they help their children with toileting.

Why are they only a problem in little girls?

Pinworms can make boys and adults itch too, especially in the anal area. Little girls have more problems because their genitourinary areas are so close to their anal areas, making them prone to "urinary" symptoms.

How do I know if it is pinworms or not?

Pinworms can sometimes be seen as threadlike, white worms in the stool or underwear. They are most likely to be found in the anal area around 11 o'clock or so at night when the female worms come out to lay their eggs. Usually they are not seen at all.

If you can't find them, how do you know whether to treat them for pinworms or not?

The itching they cause is so typical that I just prescribe Vermox based on mom's story. The entire family needs to take a single pill, and all the linens and nightclothes need to be washed. Fingernails need to be cut and toileting practices reviewed. A second pill needs to be taken again 2 weeks later.

Can you get pinworms again?

And again and again and again. There's not much you can do about it other than what you're already doing. Eventually all the toddlers in the family grow up and it's no longer a problem.

My doctor had me collect three stool samples from my little girl. It was a mess and took me 10 days just to get them to the lab. She's been itching almost 2 weeks now and we're still waiting for the final report!

Three stool samples to look for the worms or eggs is considered the "standard of care." This is very inconvenient, and often no pinworms are identified even though the child has all the symptoms.

Then what?

The Vermox is given anyway. Vermox is safe and simple and far easier than getting the three stool samples.

I've heard that you should place some Scotch tape on the anus at bedtime and then take it to the doctor the next morning. Does that help?

No, but thanks for asking.

My 8-year-old daughter doesn't complain of any burning or itching, but she urinates every 5 or 10 minutes. The doctor has checked her for UTI, external irritation, and pinworms. She's dry at night and isn't the least bit sick. I've asked him to check her for early diabetes because it runs in the family, but he just blows me off! Could she have diabetes?

Doubtful. Children with diabetes are very sick, drink and void large volumes, and wet themselves at night. Her urine would have had glucose (sugar) in it.

Then what's going on? She's driving me and her teacher crazy!

I love this word, but can never remember it and always have to look it up. It's called pollakiuria, which means frequent urination for no good reason. No one knows its cause, but most physicians who have heard of it believe that it is related to stress (we always say that when we can't figure it out). It "runs its course" in a few days to several weeks.

What should I do?

Reassure your daughter that she does not have anything seriously wrong with her and it will go away soon. Remind her that she won't have an accident if she decides to ignore the urge to urinate and waits a while before she goes to the bathroom. If you suspect that stress is contributing to the problem, you'll have to figure out how to deal with that.

Stomachache and Abdominal Pain

It's a little dangerous to offer advice about stomachache and abdominal pain in children in a book like this. Rather than leave out this very common complaint, I will reiterate that the purpose of this book is to help you understand your pediatrician's thought processes when treating your child's illnesses. It is not meant to substitute for medical care.

What's the difference between a stomachache and abdominal pain?

Nothing really to most people, but physicians use the term "stomachache" to describe the common, everyday stomach discomforts (of various causes) that children have and "abdominal pain" to describe the uncommon, occasional pain in the abdominal region that may require surgery or other significant medical intervention. This is just the pediatrician's way of communicating to other physicians (usually the surgeon) the potential seriousness of the illness, not the degree of pain (i.e., everyday stomachaches can hurt a lot, but are not serious).

When my kid gets a really bad stomachache, I always think it's serious. How can I tell if it is or not?

Don't try to make that decision; leave it to the doctor.

Are you saying that every time my kid gets a bellyache I have to take him to the doctor?

See, you've gone from "really bad stomachache" to "bellyache." You are differentiating between the degrees of pain. Either can be serious. The point is that the degree of pain is not necessarily indicative of the seriousness of the illness. It is merely one consideration.

So what's a parent to do? We're talking lots of stomachaches here.

I will list *some* of the things that a pediatrician considers when trying to determine the seriousness of abdominal complaints. They are not in order. Remember that the abdomen is not just the stomach but includes the liver, spleen, intestines, kidneys, and pancreas, to name a few of the other organs located there.

General irritability, fussiness, listlessness, distractibility
Activity level
Fever
Appetite
Change in bowel or bladder habits
Vomiting
Bleeding
Ability or willingness to walk, move, climb, sit up
Weight changes
Duration, severity, nature of pain
Night pain
Other associated symptoms not necessarily related to the abdomen
Family, school, and social considerations

Can't you tell just by "checking him"?

No. The physical examination is important in determining the seriousness of the complaint, but, again, it is only one part of the big picture.

What about blood tests or x-rays?

These provide additional information in suspicious situations, but they can still be normal even if the situation is serious.

Isn't there some simple way to know when you should begin to worry?

Not really. However, stomachaches are common and serious illness is not. There is usually time to wait and see how things are going before you race off to the doctor. Time frequently sorts things out and, at the very least, offers the doctor more to go on when you do decide it's time to get your child checked out.

What if he needs emergency surgery for something like appendicitis? That can't wait, can it?

Not for long, but fortunately *in urgent situations* the symptoms correlate pretty well with the degree of urgency. In other words, a child with appendicitis who isn't that sick yet has fewer symptoms and more time than a very ill child with a lot of symptoms who needs to have surgery right away. A parent usually doesn't have trouble recognizing a serious illness. They have more trouble acknowledging that their child just has a bad gas problem.

I worry more about cancer or a tumor or something.

That is a possibility. However, the diagnosis of that type of problem is not usually made in a single office visit or after a couple of complaints of stomachache. It is reasonable to wait and see how things pan out over a period of time before investigating every stomachache.

How long?

It really depends on a lot of things, some of which were listed earlier. Days to months sometimes.

What do I do in the meantime?

Your doctor usually has some simple suggestions on what to do for specific symptoms during the wait and see period. The odds are always in favor of the pain resolving on its own or declaring itself more specifically as time goes by.

In summary, abdominal pain in children can be tricky business and shouldn't be taken lightly. However, a parent's judgment is usually good enough when it really matters, such as in surgical emergencies. Most other complaints can be investigated methodically over a period of time (hours to months) until the cause is found or they go away.

Nosebleeds

Nosebleeds are extremely common in healthy children. The nose is full of tiny blood vessels that are vulnerable to scratching and picking. Unless associated with other symptoms (bleeding elsewhere, bruising, fevers, weight loss, and decreased appetite), nosebleeds in and of themselves are not of concern to the pediatrician.

My son's nose bleeds almost every night for weeks! Is that normal?

Once a nose bleeds it is likely to bleed again. The dried blood in the nose can be itchy and kids will rub and pick more. The fragile blood vessels of the nose never have a chance to heal completely before they are disturbed again.

Nosebleeds are most common in the cold, dry months when heaters are on. This dries out the mucous membranes of the nose and makes them more fragile. It is also the time for colds, and kids are constantly rubbing and picking at their noses. It's a perfect setting for frequent nosebleeds.

But it can't be good for him. Isn't there something I can do?

To prevent frequent nosebleeds, keep your child's hands clean and his nails cut. Try to teach him to leave his nose alone and use a Kleenex (yeah right!). Run a humidifier in his room, and place some Vaseline or greasy antibiotic ointment into his nostrils at bedtime.

Shouldn't we check the blood count or something?

It is extremely rare to have an abnormal blood count from frequent nosebleeds. A blood count is necessary only if there are other signs and symptoms of illness that are of concern to the doctor.

Head Lice

Head lice infestation is a common problem in preschool and school-age children. It is caused by a louse (small bug) that makes its home on the human scalp and lays its eggs, called nits, on individual hairs. Head lice affect 8 to 12 million children a year. This is a contagious disease and *not* a result of poor hygiene.

If it's not caused by poor hygiene, how come some kids get it and others don't?

For the same reasons some kids get ear infections and some don't. Everyone is susceptible, but some people are more prone than others. Although I haven't read any studies (I don't think there are any) on which types of hair are more prone to infestation, in my experience the *texture* of the hair seems to play as much a role as the length of the hair. Some hair seems to be "slick" and more challenging to lice, and some hair seems to be more coarse and accommodating to lice. It's also harder to see head lice in blonde or thick-haired kids even if present.

Does having long hair make a child more susceptible?

Theoretically no, but realistically yes. What this means is that lice infest the *scalp*, not hair, but long hair makes it easier for the lice to get to the scalp in the first place and set up housekeeping—long-haired kids do get more head lice. In addition, if long-haired children spend more time combing and "fixing" their hair, there is more opportunity for infected stray hairs to be strewn about the environment. Short-haired children can become infested just as easily when their scalps contact infested hairs, but that happens less often because they have less hair.

Can't they get head lice from the dog or stuffed animals?

No, the head louse can only survive and reproduce in humans.

Then why do we have to bag all the stuffed animals and "sterilize" all the sheets and pajamas and stuff?

Good question. Human hairs fall out with the unhatched nits (eggs) attached to them. If a human scalp comes near enough to a nit near the time of hatching, the newborn louse can make its way to its next victim and a new infestation occurs. However, a louse cannot survive off a human scalp for very long, probably only a few hours. A louse that doesn't find a home soon after hatching dies quickly. Any item that has the potential to harbor "loose" human hairs with attached nits must be washed properly or placed in plastic bags until all the nits are hatched and the lice are dead.

We've religiously followed the shampooing, NIX* application, and nit removal techniques and washed and bagged everything, but we still can't get rid of them! What's the problem?

It only takes one stray hair with a nit on it to attach itself near a human scalp to start the whole process over again. Human hairs fall out regularly all over the place and kids' heads are everywhere.

I thought that the NIX creme conditioner was supposed to prevent reinfestation for up to 2 weeks. Shouldn't all the nits have hatched and lice have died by then?

Yes, they should have. If the medication adequately prevented reinfestation for 2 weeks, that should be enough time for all the nits to hatch and the lice to die. There are several reasons for the reinfestation: The lice may be developing some resistance to the medication. It's difficult to coat every single hair on a head (especially in uncooperative children and large families) and wash or isolate every potential hair/nit hangout. Moms frequently start vigorously shampooing every night and washing off all the applied medication that's meant to last for 2 weeks. In addition, it's hard to see lice and nits in thick-haired or blonde kids and unrecognized infestation may not get treated. There's a ready supply of new head lice whenever children are in close quarters.

What else can we do?

Some people forget to towel dry the hair before putting on the NIX. This can cause some dilution of the medication and it doesn't adhere to the hair like it should. It's also important to shampoo the hair first and *not* use anything with a conditioner in it because that can "coat" the hair and prevent the medication from "sticking." If you can stand it, *avoid reshampooing* the hair for as long as you can (several days at least) since this can remove the NIX residue from the hair. Keeping long hair braided or tied in such a way as to minimize contact with nits or lice can also help prevent reinfestation.

---

*A medicated creme hair conditioner.

Can I use the medication again?

You can reuse the medication after 1 week. Try even harder this time to coat the scalp, cover every single hair, remove every nit, and get all the stray hairs in your house.

Can I use the medication on my baby?

No. It is not approved for infants under 2 months because its safety in this age group has not been investigated yet. However, most young infants have such a small amount of fine, thin hair that lice can't grab hold of it and make it to the scalp. Nits don't "stick" that well. If your baby does have lice or nits, manual removal should be fairly simple.

Will fumigation by the pest control people help?

No.

I know you said that we can't get lice from our cat and dog, but couldn't some of our hairs end up on them if they sleep in our beds?

Yes, there is some risk of this reinfesting you, but not in infesting your pets. The human head louse can survive only on human scalp. Bag your dog and cat or brush and wash them well and keep them away from the living quarters as long as you can.

I've done all that, and this is the third time this year my kids have gotten head lice from school. It's impossible!

It is impossible without the cooperation of the entire school. When there is an outbreak of head lice in a school, all infested individuals and their potential contacts need to be thoroughly treated and their environments meticulously deloused. But, most important of all, everyone needs to be treated at the same time and not allowed to return to school without a careful check by someone who knows what she's doing. At our school trained mother volunteers stand at the entrance to the school and carefully check every single head. No one gets in with lice or nits. We also need to develop some more medications.

Poison Ivy and Oak

Poison ivy and oak produce oils that irritate skin on contact. This results in localized redness, swelling, and itching where the oil touches the skin. Once the oil is washed off, the reaction will subside in a couple of days.

People who are *allergic* to poison ivy or oak (and many people are) will have a more severe local reaction and additional reactions distant from the site of contact can occur.

Why is there a rash in places such as the stomach that didn't come in contact with the oils? Was it spread by scratching or a second contact with the plants?

No. It is not the result of scratching and rubbing or a second contact. The rash, itching, and swelling are systemic manifestations of allergy that were set in motion at the time of original contact. Of course, additional contact with the plants will aggravate the problem.

Can you "catch" poison ivy from someone else?

No. You cannot "catch" poison ivy or oak from other people or animals unless they still have oil on their skin (or hair or clothes).

My son was around poison ivy last week, but he didn't get a rash until today. Is the rash from the poison ivy or something else?

The rash from poison ivy frequently takes several days to develop. It may not peak until a week or so after the initial exposure.

My son was exposed to poison ivy over the weekend. It's been over a week and it's still spreading and seems to be getting worse. Is it because he keeps scratching?

No, scratching will not spread poison ivy, but it may add fuel to the allergic fire. It can also lead to infection down the line.

How long is it supposed to last?

Symptoms can come and go for weeks and then return after they seemingly have resolved.

What can I do?

Since the allergic reaction can come and go for weeks even with no additional contact with the plant, treatment depends on where you are in the time course of the reaction as well as its severity. For mild cases, oral Benadryl is usually adequate. Topical hydrocortisone cream can relieve *localized* itching. For moderate to severe cases, oral steroids may be necessary to make the patient comfortable.

Animal Bites and Rabies

CATS

All bites by cats are puncture wounds and should be cleaned out with soap and water and examined by a doctor within 24 hours or so. Bites to the face or scalp should be examined as soon as possible (within hours).

If it's not during regular office hours, is it really necessary to go to the emergency department?

I would. The wound can be cleansed more thoroughly, antibiotics can be prescribed, and a tetanus shot given if necessary. The proper authorities can also be notified of the animal bite.

Are antibiotics always necessary?

Generally, yes. Antibiotics are recommended for all cat bites because of the depth of penetration. Deep wounds pose a greater risk of infection and cannot drain or be observed easily. One in three cat bites becomes infected.

If your child's tetanus shot is up to date, is it necessary to get one?

Probably not, but even if the tetanus shot is current, an additional shot may still be recommended in some situations and it can be given in the emergency department.

Why are cat bites so worrisome?

Cat germs are no more dangerous, they are just injected more deeply into the tissues.

DOGS

Dog bites are usually shallow and wide and easier to clean out and to observe for infection. They are not *routinely* treated with antibiotics.

Do I need to go to the emergency department for an ordinary dog bite?

Not usually. They can be handled at home unless they are on the face or scalp or are particularly deep or large. Some wounds may need to be stitched for a better cosmetic result. If your child's tetanus shot is current, you can check with your doctor in a day or so to see if an additional one is recommended.

RABIES

All *mammals* can be infected with rabies. Rabies still occurs in this country and is always fatal.

What exactly is rabies?

It is a virus that travels via the nervous system from the area of the bite to the brain where it causes death.

Are pets at risk?

Domestic cats and dogs are at low risk if their rabies shots are current and they are not in contact with any wild or stray animals. All bites should still be checked out thoroughly to be sure.

Is a bite necessary to transmit rabies?

No. The virus can be transmitted if the infectious secretions of a rabid animal contact a break in the skin or a mucous membrane (eyes, nose, or mouth). Because of this, *any* contact between children and stray or wild mammals should be investigated whether they were actually bitten or not. It is important to notify the proper authorities in your community. Rabies prophylaxis may be indicated in some situations.

Is prevention still 20 shots in the stomach?

No. It's not that bad anymore. Now it's four or five spread out over several weeks, and they can be given in the traditional sites.

Warts

Warts are common in healthy children. They are caused by a virus and like all viruses will run their course in time. Warts tend to run in families and are easily spread to other family members.

How long does it take a wart to run its course?

Warts can take from 9 months to 2 years or so to go away. Warts are frequently multiple and in different stages of resolution in different parts of the body.

What is the best treatment for warts?

There is no single treatment for warts that is satisfactory for everyone. It depends on the age of the child and the size, location, and number of warts. Here are some general guidelines:

1. Single warts that are not bothersome to the child should be left alone and they will go away on their own in time.
2. A wart that is in a location that is particularly unsightly or prone to trauma (fingers and hand) should be removed by the dermatologist when convenient.
3. A plantar wart (one found on the bottom of the foot) starts out as a tiny pinhead sized black speck. It grows slowly into a very painful deep wart. Kids don't usually notice until they have pain when they walk. The best thing to do is see the dermatologist for quick removal as soon as possible. They'll usually "work you in."

Can't I just remove that one little wart at home with that stuff you get at the drugstore?

Sure you can. Home remedies contain the same chemicals used in the pediatrician's office. They still take at least a couple of months to work and a lot of cooperation from the parent and child. Good luck, you'll need it. I don't think it's worth it for a simple wart.

I think I'll just wait and see if it goes away on its own. What do you think?

Good idea. Wait to remove a single wart that is not bothersome since it is likely that others may pop up as time goes by. Once several have accumulated and become particularly bothersome, a trip to the dermatologist may be worthwhile. The whole family can go!

It seems like a lot of trouble and expense to go to the dermatologist for a wart.

You're right it is, but so are those home remedies.

What will the dermatologist do?

Dermatologists have several options for removing warts, including toxic chemicals, freezing, burning, cutting, and scraping. The method they choose depends on the age of the child and the size, location, and number of warts to be removed. Most can be completely removed in one or two sessions.

That sounds terrible. Does it hurt?

Dermatologists are really good at it and it shouldn't hurt. It beats the couple of months and cooperation that it takes to paint on chemicals at home or the pediatrician's office. For warts, I would just skip the drugstore and pediatrician altogether and go straight to the dermatologist.

Poisoning

In emergency poisoning situations syrup of ipecac was the mainstay of treatment for decades. In the past few years ipecac to induce vomiting has lost favor with the poison control people. The problems with ipecac were many, primarily remembering the long list of things that you were *not* supposed to use ipecac for. By the time the poisoning was discovered and the decision to give ipecac was made, it was too late to gain any benefit from vomiting.

Should I throw out my bottle of syrup of ipecac?

No. Ipecac is still useful when a poisoning is discovered immediately and is due to something on the "okay" list. Be sure to use the right dose (check the bottle) and follow it with plenty of water. The poison control center should still be called as soon as possible for further instructions.

What if the label on the bottle says it expired last year?

Ipecac is good for up to 4 years after the expiration date.

If it's too late for vomiting to help, how do you get rid of the poison?

In most cases of poisoning, activated charcoal is now given to the child to swallow (or is put into the stomach via a flexible plastic tube). Most poisons will stick to the charcoal. A cathartic can then be administered orally to wash the whole thing out.

What should I do if I discover my baby has gotten into something that may be poisonous?

Call poison control. Keep the poison control number on the phone and make sure that everyone in the house knows it is there.

What if I find that my child got into something but it's been a while and he seems all right to me?

If there has been a delay in discovering the poisoning, call poison control *first* (before giving ipecac) and be prepared to go to the emergency department immediately if instructed to do so. Many substances have delayed effects, and one of the most important aspects of poison management is careful observation and monitoring of the patient until the danger has passed. There are some antidotes and other supportive therapies for poisonings that may be useful.

What are some of the most common poisoning agents in children?

Fortunately, education and the cooperation of industry are making it harder for kids to hurt themselves when they do get into potentially poisonous substances. There is a decrease in serious poisoning incidents, especially in the home. Lock up the prenatal vitamins, the dishwasher detergent, and grandma's purse. Outside the house we still see problems with pesticides and occasionally with other products found in the garage that are just thoughtlessly made available to curious kids.

Cuts and Stitches

Any wound will heal more quickly with less scarring if it is stitched. However, depending on the size and location of the cut, it may or may not be worth the trouble of going to the emergency department or doctor's office for stitching.

How can I tell for sure if my child needs stitches or not?

If you aren't sure whether it is worth it or not, it is okay to wait a day or two and see what happens. If the cut is healing and is not in an area where it is likely to be reinjured, there's no need for stitches. If the cut is not healing, usually because of repetitive trauma, it can still be stitched.

Are there any cuts that should *always* be stitched?

It's a good idea to have a cut on the face stitched as soon as possible for a better cosmetic result and on the extremities where there is a lot of motion or risk for reinjury.

My daughter just cut her face and I can't tell if she needs stitches or not. What should I do?

All cuts will heal faster and better if sutured properly. Any cut (not scratch) on the face should be handled by a plastic surgeon if available or a general surgeon if one is not.

I don't know any surgeons. Won't my pediatrician do?

Pediatricians in a busy office don't usually have time to do this. They get out of practice and should not attempt to stitch up facial cuts. A butterfly bandage may be adequate for a very small or one that is in a concealed area (chin), and the pediatrician can apply this. Call first to make sure you won't be in a crowded waiting room with a lot of sick kids. (I wouldn't want him stitching up my kid's chin under those circumstances.) When in doubt, see the surgeon and save yourself a trip. Make sure your child's tetanus shot is up to date.

My son cut his hand a couple of days ago. It wasn't very bad and he bandaged it himself, but it keeps opening up again. Is it too late for stitches?

I wish I knew where it was written that "it's too late for stitches when. . . ." I hear that all the time and it's just not true. Any wound can be stitched by a surgeon. If the wound is already healing well, there's no reason to have it stitched, but then you wouldn't be asking, would you? If it keeps opening up or bleeding or oozing, it is not healing well and it needs to be cleaned out (debrided) by a surgeon and stitched. Check with the pediatrician on your child's tetanus status.

Bed-Wetting

Bed-wetting is a frustrating and unnerving problem for parents and children alike, but there's not much that can be done about it. It has a very strong hereditary component, especially in boys. It is attributed to small bladder capacity and unusually deep sleep, but no one really knows for sure why older children still wet their beds.

What age should my child be before I do something about the bed-wetting?

At 7 years or so in girls and 9 years or so in boys. Before then, it is best just to limit fluid intake at dinner and have the child get up at least once during the night to urinate, usually right before the parents go to bed.

Should I expect him to clean up after himself?

It's not his fault and he should not be punished—he's embarrassed enough as it is. It is reasonable to expect him to help out with the laundry because he's old enough to. Work out a system for dealing with the sheets and pajamas that is agreeable to everyone.

What about alarms?

For older kids, an alarm clock can help awaken them to go to the bathroom a couple of times a night. Bed-wetting alarms sold in drugstores are supposed to be 70% effective in controlling bed-wetting. They arouse the child as soon as they sense wet underwear. They are worth a try in older motivated, cooperative children.

What about medication?

Medications such as imipramine (an antidepressant medication that promotes urinary retention as a side effect) work about half the time, have a lot of side effects, and are extremely dangerous if overdosed. Bed-wetting recurs when the medication is stopped.

What about that new nasal spray?

The new drug is DDAVP nasal spray and it is expensive. This is a hormone that actually decreases the amount of urine produced during the night when taken at bedtime.

Are there any side effects?

The child has to be careful about drinking too much water in the evening, but this is usually not a problem for bed-wetters.

How well does it work?

DDAVP works better for children who are just about to outgrow bed-wetting anyway and offers temporary relief during overnighters or summer camp. It can make a big difference in the quality of life of an older bed-wetter.

Does the bed-wetting recur when the medication is stopped?

Yes, unless the child outgrew his problem during the time he was on the medication. This accounts for the variable success and relapse rate.

What's the best approach?

Patience, support, and understanding with the occasional use of DDAVP or imipramine for special occasions or to give everyone a much needed break.

Attention Deficit/Hyperactivity Disorder

The concept of attention deficit/hyperactivity disorder (AD/HD) is not new. In the past "minimal brain dysfunction" was the scientific term used to describe isolated, discrete problems in brain function in an otherwise healthy child. Careful neurologic testing, however, usually revealed other subtle problems in brain function.

What is AD/HD?

AD/HD is a brain dysfunction marked by a short attention span and/or hyperactivity and impulsivity. Therefore a child can have AD/HD and not have an attention problem at all or he can sit still as a statue and not pay attention to a word you say or do a minute's worth of work.

Why don't they just call it two separate problems?

Since it is likely that different parts of the brain are responsible for these dysfunctions, I don't know why the experts don't classify them as different problems and then note that it is common to have both. Old traditions die hard I guess.

My son's teacher thinks that he has AD/HD. How does she know?

Although there is no doubt that the condition is grossly overdiagnosed, there are some children whose attention spans and/or activity levels fall at the extreme ends of the bell curve. Whether this is called a disease or not has to be determined on an individual basis.

What do you mean by that?

For example, the shortest kids in the school may come from short families (i.e., there's nothing wrong with them) or because they have undiagnosed kidney disease. An experienced schoolteacher may or may not be capable of determining which children have a real medical condition.

He's not doing as well this year, but he doesn't like his teacher. Wouldn't that explain a lot?

It might. One of the most difficult aspects of diagnosing AD/HD involves sorting out the secondary behaviors that children develop because of their primary problem of attention deficit or hyperactivity and impulsivity. When children don't meet others' expectations, their feelings of inadequacy can become so overpowering that additional maladaptive behaviors develop, such as rage, violence, apathy, or insubordination. It doesn't take long for a simple attention problem to become a big behavioral problem.

How do you figure it out?

Unfortunately, these children are not identified until they have a multitude of problems, and it is very difficult to untangle them and get to the source of the problem. It may be impossible.

Can't you run some tests or something?

No. There's no blood test or brain scan that will identify these kids (yet). Therefore many "difficult" children are labeled as having AD/HD and placed on stimulant medications such as Ritalin.

What is Ritalin and does it work?

Ritalin is an amphetamine that will make anyone perform better on certain tasks in the short term, just like the caffeine punch in a cup of coffee in the morning increases performance. This short-term "real" improvement combined with the very powerful placebo effect has added to the popularity of medication for difficult children. It doesn't take too long, however, for most parents giving twice-daily medication to sour on the whole thing.

Are there any good data on Ritalin's effectiveness?

Ritalin has been given to all kinds of "difficult" kids who may or may not have met the ever-changing criteria for a diagnosis of AD/HD. The response has been variable and unpredictable. It is impossible to scientifically evaluate the effectiveness of medication for AD/HD until there is a way to scientifically identify the kids who actually have AD/HD. It might not even be a single disease.

How can you tell if my child's behavior is due to AD/HD or something else?

You can't. The diagnosis of AD/HD is made after ruling out (to the best of everyone's ability) other causes of his "poor" behavior. Unfortunately, these other common causes such as learning disability, inconsistent parenting, emotional problems, or mental illness are just as nebulous as AD/HD.

How is the diagnosis made?

A checklist of behaviors that have been present for a period of time are used to make the diagnosis. Parents and teachers have more insight into the child than the doctor, and treatment is often instituted based primarily on interviews with the parents and teachers.

Prescribing stimulant medication and life-altering therapies on such subjective, biased information can't be good, but right now that's all we've got.

My son meets all the criteria for AD/HD and is doing much better with medication. Is there anything else I should be doing?

For those children who are "correctly" identified as having a primary brain problem with attention deficit or hyperactivity/impulsivity, a combined approach using behavioral, environmental, and medicinal therapies is more successful in producing sustained improvement.

Will he outgrow his behavior problems?

Primary brain problems are not outgrown, and the support offered to these children should not be abruptly terminated just because they grow up.

Heart Murmurs

Heart murmurs are the result of blood flowing through the heart and its vessels—they can be normal or abnormal.

What is a normal heart murmur?

The chest walls of children are relatively thin, and blood flowing through the heart can frequently be heard in healthy children with perfect hearts. These murmurs are referred to as innocent, functional, or normal.

When do you hear innocent murmurs?

Is that a trick question? Always. If you can't hear it, it's not a murmur is it? An innocent murmur can be heard at anytime. Many innocent murmurs are not heard except during illness when the heart is working harder than usual.

Will my daughter outgrow it?

Innocent murmurs may or may not be heard as the child grows bigger; it doesn't matter one way or the other.

If it is normal, why is it even noted at all?

Good question. Many pediatricians don't say anything about it at all, but most make a note of it in the chart. No one wants to be accused of not noticing it.

My daughter saw a different doctor while we were on vacation and he heard a heart murmur. I was really worried since my pediatrician had never mentioned it before. Why didn't he tell me?

He didn't want you to worry. This is a good reason for pediatricians to tell patients about innocent murmurs. In addition, it helps other doctors to know that it had been heard in the past.

Grandma took my son to her doctor while I was out of town. He heard a heart murmur and ordered a chest x-ray film and an ECG! Was all this necessary?

What, no treadmill? Adult doctors aren't used to hearing them.

What's an abnormal murmur?

Abnormal heart murmurs are caused by turbulent blood flow through abnormal hearts and vessels. Some are minor and some are very serious.

Can the pediatrician tell the difference?

I certainly hope so. Most pediatricians can tell which murmurs are of concern and require a referral to the cardiologist and which are innocent. If there is any doubt, pediatricians refer. I'm sure cardiologists get tired of us sending them patients with innocent murmurs, but better safe than sorry.

I took my 3-year-old in to the doctor's office for a cold and my pediatrician heard a heart murmur that he'd never heard before. He thinks it's innocent but isn't sure and wants to recheck him in a couple of weeks. If he doesn't know now, how will he know then? Shouldn't I just see the cardiologist?

If your child is already 3 years old and has no signs or symptoms of heart disease, it is extremely unlikely that he has any significant abnormalities that couldn't wait another couple of weeks. It is very likely that your child's heart murmur was heard because he was sick when you brought him in. He'll be well in a couple of weeks and the murmur may no longer be there. Murmurs due to heart disease do not go away on their own. If the murmur is still present and the pediatrician cannot be absolutely sure it is innocent, he will refer you at that point.

7

Immunizations

The immunization schedule for children becomes more complex yearly. New vaccines are added, old ones are revised, and there are always several more changes on the horizon.

There are so many changes it worries me that they're rushing things and not taking the time to see if it's the right thing?

It may seem that all the changes cannot possibly be well thought out, but let me assure you that this is not the case. Many of the "new" changes in immunizations are only new in the United States. Canada, Europe, and Japan are well ahead of us in implementing changes, and often changes in this country are based on the years (sometimes decades) of experience in other countries.

It's hard and expensive to keep up with all these shots for diseases I've never even heard of. Can't we relax a little bit?

The reason you've never heard of these diseases is because of the diligence of others before you. The overwhelming success of immunizations have ironically led to their own downfall. Vaccines have eliminated so many of the serious infections of childhood that parents of young children today have no idea how bad things were before the age of immunization. Many have become complacent about getting their children immunized.

It makes me nervous injecting all these dangerous things into my baby. Am I wrong?

Like everything in life, no vaccine is perfect, but the risks from immunization are infinitesimal compared with the risks of natural infection. However, since most people these days have no experience with natural infection, it is often hard to make this argument. I wonder how many people would refuse a vaccine for childhood cancer or AIDS?

Can't some of the vaccines actually cause the illness?

Vaccines are classified as either "killed" or "live, attenuated." Killed vaccines cannot induce any form of the illness they are designed to prevent. Live, attenuated vaccines are actually weakened versions of the infectious agent and by definition cause a mild (hopefully unrecognized) form of the disease.

Why not just use killed vaccines rather than taking a chance with the live ones?

Killed vaccines are less effective overall than live vaccines in preventing disease, and their protective effects don't last as long as live vaccines. That is why so many booster doses of killed vaccines are required for successful immunization. If we had to rely on people to get frequent injections of a vaccine, there would be a lot of inadequately immunized individuals and therefore a lot more disease.

If live vaccines actually "cause" illness, why not just take my chances with these rare diseases?

The reason that a live vaccine for an illness was developed in the first place was that the disease was very serious. There's a vaccine for polio but not one for the common cold. The "illness" induced by a live vaccine goes unrecognized most of the time and only causes mild symptoms occasionally. With a vaccine, you pick and choose the time when you are going to expose your child to the very mild form of the disease as opposed to the random attack of a more virulent infection.

Aren't live vaccines dangerous for people with cancer or other medical problems?

Caution is necessary in children who are immunocompromised or are in contact with someone who is immunocompromised. The danger must be weighed against the risk of natural infection.

Why do vaccines have so many side effects?

The only consistent side effect of vaccination is tenderness at the site where the needle penetrated the skin. The purpose of a vaccine is to activate the immune system, which causes an inflammatory response that subsequently protects the body from future infection. The so-called side effects of a vaccine are the direct result of successful immunization.

Sometimes my doctor gives four or five vaccinations at a time. Is it safe to give so many at the same time?

Medically speaking, it is safe and effective to administer many vaccinations concurrently. There are a couple of exceptions and every pediatrician is aware of them. There is disagreement among pediatricians, family physicians, and parents, however, on the emotional impact of multiple injections on a child. Surprisingly, parents are more apt to want to "get it over with" than physicians. Remember that even a single injection of combination vaccines such as diphtheria, pertussis, and tetanus (DPT) or measles, mumps, and rubella (MMR) provokes an immune response to multiple disease-causing agents.

I've heard that all these childhood immunizations could lead to chronic diseases in later years. Is this possible?

The diseases for which vaccines are available are known to result in death or significant disability in most cases (that is why a vaccine was developed in the first place). There is no evidence that sparing children serious disease through immunization will make them susceptible to chronic illness later in life. Would you rather sacrifice some children on the off chance that those who survive to adulthood will be ensured of good health?

I don't have any problems with the old vaccines, but I'm really concerned about all these new ones.

You're not alone. New vaccines always give rise to suspicion and doubt. The ones that were such a big deal 10 years ago (pertussis vaccine, for example) are hardly even mentioned anymore. People forget what all the hoopla was about.

I admit that most of my concern stems from horror stories I've heard on TV lately, but aren't they just reporting the facts?

They try to report the scientific facts as *they* understand them and then translate them to a diverse audience. I know how much miscommunication can occur in a one-on-one conversation in my small office (that's why I wrote this book), so it is no surprise to me to see how much misinformation there is in the press. The intentions are sincere, but it is difficult to comprehend the whole story and then tell it in 5 or 10 minutes.

I'm sorry, but I just don't like the idea of vaccines. Why should I have my child get them to go to school if I don't want to? What business is it of theirs?

It is very important to vaccinate *all* children who can be successfully immunized to protect the children who cannot be immunized because of legitimate medical reasons. The children who cannot take the vaccines depend on the principle of "herd immunity" to protect them from disease.

What's "herd immunity"?

A principle of immunity that states that even if you cannot successfully vaccinate *all* the individuals in a population ("herd"), enough can be vaccinated to prevent the disease from infecting those who cannot be successfully vaccinated for whatever reason.

How does that work? If someone can't be immunized and the disease is still around, why won't he catch it?

He can, but the risk is low. Herd immunity acknowledges the fact that at best a single vaccine is around 90% effective in preventing an individual from getting a disease. "Booster" doses can push this number up closer to 100%, but it's never perfect.

In the rare event that an individual's vaccine does not "take" and he catches the disease, the chances of him coming into close contact with another susceptible individual is slim. The disease stops with that individual if there's no one around to give it to. There will always be some isolated cases, but major epidemics are rare.

Is it true that even if a vaccine "fails" and you get sick, that it is a milder case?

Yes.

I know they've eradicated smallpox and are coming close with polio. Any others?

The goal of mass immunization is always disease eradication, but so far that has only happened with smallpox.

How can we eradicate other diseases?

If everyone eligible received all the recommended vaccines, many more infectious diseases could be eliminated. This would protect the others who cannot be immunized for whatever reason (e.g., fetuses, children with cancer, and pregnant women).

I think that immunizations are great! Are there any others that aren't on the required list that I can get?

Yes. There are a couple of others readily available on request—those for hepatitis A, influenza, and pneumococcal pneumonia.

Influenza vaccines, polio vaccines, chickenpox vaccine, and hepatitis vaccines are some of the most commonly misunderstood and I will discuss them separately. Questions about the others are addressed under "Miscellaneous Immunization Questions."

Polio Vaccine

Two vaccines are available for polio. Both were discovered at approximately the same time in the 1950s. It has made polio virtually unheard of in this country. There is the killed injected polio vaccine (IPV) and the live, attenuated oral polio vaccine (OPV). As far as inducing immunity, the live OPV is more effective than the killed IPV.

If the vaccines have been around for so long, why is there currently so much debate about IPV and OPV?

In the United States the OPV has been used almost exclusively for decades with great success. The only drawback is that it causes about seven cases of polio a year. When natural poliovirus was still around, this was considered an acceptable trade-off. Now that there is no natural poliovirus in this country, it is no longer acceptable to have vaccine-induced cases. Changing from OPV to IPV is now being considered.

If IPV doesn't cause any cases of polio, why don't they just use it?

It's not that simple. IPV has to be injected. People are resistant to more shots, especially since we have an oral vaccine that works better. Much of the early success of OPV was because it could be handed out in sugar cubes at malls.

Since IPV is a killed virus, it is not as effective as OPV and more booster shots are required. For these reasons, more people will be susceptible to polio than they were with OPV, and there may be an increase in the number of *natural* polio cases. It doesn't make any sense to eliminate the seven vaccine-induced cases only to replace them with an even greater number of *wild* (natural) polio cases.

Natural polio hasn't been found in this country for years. How can anybody get it?

Many countries in the world still have epidemics of natural polio. People come and people go.

So what's going to happen?

There's still a lot of debate, but it looks as if the new recommendation will be two doses of injected IPV, followed by two doses of OPV.

Will this solve all the problems?

Everyone hopes so. The theory is that the two injections of IPV will confer enough immunity in young infants to prevent any cases of polio that the subsequent two doses of OPV might cause. It is hoped that herd immunity will confer enough protection for those young infants receiving the less effective IPV. It's all theoretical at this point and only time will tell. Fortunately, other countries around the world are ahead of us in dealing with this problem and we are learning from them.

Influenza Vaccine

Influenza is a moderate to severe respiratory infection characterized by fever that lasts 5 to 10 days, cough or chest discomfort, fatigue, and generalized aches. It can last up to 10 to 14 days. It is not a bad cold or a stomach virus.

There are many strains of influenza virus that basically can be classified as types A or B. Influenza viruses are epidemic in the cold weather months, and although not life threatening to otherwise healthy adults and children, they can be fatal to immunocompromised persons or those with underlying conditions such as heart or lung disease.

Every year an influenza vaccine is prepared using the three most likely viral strains to circulate and cause epidemic influenza. A yearly vaccination is the best way to avoid becoming ill with influenza.

My doctor says that only certain high-risk people need to be immunized?

Anyone who doesn't want to suffer from flu symptoms can be immunized. Infants as young as 6 months can receive the vaccine for influenza. It is strongly recommended for high-risk people since they are the ones most likely to suffer life-threatening complications.

I've had flu shots several times in the past. Why do I have to keep getting them?

Each year scientists predict which influenza strains are most likely to circulate and they specifically develop a vaccine for these strains. Your previous vaccines may or may not have contained the current year's strains. Protection wanes over time (months generally) since it is a killed rather than a live vaccine. Over the years, however, you will start to build up a longer lasting immunity to many common strains.

What if they are wrong and the wrong strains are used in the vaccine?

In the last couple of decades they have rarely been incorrect. When they are, there is a lot more flu. Yearly immunization offers some protection during the occasional "off" year.

Are there any side effects?

Like all vaccines, there can be some mild local tenderness at the site of injection.

Is one shot enough to prevent the flu?

First-time vaccine recipients must receive two injections 1 month apart. After that, one shot a year is sufficient. The vaccine should offer protection within 2 to 4 weeks and last throughout the season.

I know a lot of people who say that the flu shot gave them the flu. Is this possible?

Since many people don't know the difference between a bad cold and influenza, it is a popular misconception that the vaccine can cause the flu. This is not true. The vaccine is prepared from killed viruses and cannot cause influenza, but it does take a couple of weeks to confer immunity and you could come down with flu in the interim.

I know some people who got the flu anyway.

No vaccine is perfect, but when vaccinated persons develop influenza, the symptoms are much milder than they would have been otherwise. (How are you so sure it was influenza?)

I've always been good about getting my flu shot, but missed it this year. Is that okay?

Those who receive yearly injections are at decreased risk of developing influenza even if they miss a year or if the vaccine doesn't incorporate the correct strains. Influenza strains share many similarities, and the vaccines of all the previous years can add up to offer some protection. I wouldn't depend on this, however, if you really want to avoid influenza infection.

Isn't there a medication to prevent influenza now?

The antiviral medication Flumadine can be used to prevent influenza A but not type B in unvaccinated persons or while waiting for the vaccine to "kick in." Daily medication for months is not as good as receiving the vaccine for the prevention of illness.

Chickenpox Vaccine

The chickenpox vaccine (Varivax) is now routinely recommended for children 12 to 18 months of age and for those over the age of 12 years who have not had chickenpox. It can be given at any age after the age of 12 months. It is hoped that it will soon be incorporated in the MMR shot or other combination vaccine.

I heard that Varivax can cause chickenpox.

It is a live, attenuated vaccine and has the potential of causing a mild, usually unrecognized illness up to 1 month after vaccination.

Are there any side effects?

Like all vaccines, it can cause a mild local reaction at the injection site.

Can it be given to children who live with immunocompromised people?

As with all live vaccines, caution must be used when administering the vaccine to immunocompromised persons or those who share a household with such persons. Almost always the vaccine can be given safely.

Can my child receive the vaccine if I am pregnant?

There is no danger to pregnant women who have already had chickenpox or to their fetus, but there is a theoretical risk to newborns. It should be remembered, however, that a susceptible pregnant worman and her fetus are at much more significant risk if exposed to the ever-present natural virus.

I've never had chickenpox and i'm pregnant. Can I get the vaccine?

No. The vaccine is not recommended during pregnancy even though you and your fetus are at greater risk from natural chickenpox infection.

I have two toddlers who haven't had chickenpox. Wouldn't it be a lot worse for me and my unborn baby if we caught it from them than from the vaccine?

Probably, but no one knows for sure and no physician wants to take the blame if something bad happens. It's not anybody's fault if you acquire chickenpox naturally.

Is there anything I can do?

Have your toddlers immunized as soon as possible.

I'm not sure if my child had chickenpox or not. He had a couple of spots that looked like mosquito bites. What should I do?

It won't hurt to immunize him anyway if you aren't sure whether he has had it or not.

I'm not sure if I've had chickenpox, and I am trying to get pregnant. Is there anything I can do?

You can either postpone trying to get pregnant a couple of months and get immunized or you can have a blood test to check to see if you've actually had chickenpox and then get immunized if necessary.

How effective is the vaccine?

The vaccine is believed to be around 85% protective, and those that do become symptomatic have a very mild illness.

Can it increase the risk for shingles?

There is no increased incidence of shingles in vaccine recipients, and the evidence suggests that the incidence of shingles may actually be less in immunized people as compared with those who suffer natural chickenpox infection.

Isn't there a medication for chickenpox now?

Yes. It's called acyclovir and it can help reduce the symptoms if started within 24 hours of the onset of the rash. Vaccination is much better.

How many shots do you need?

Currently only one injection is needed in young children and two injections at least 1 month apart in those over the age of 12 years. At this time no additional boosters are recommended.

What if it is decided that you need to get a second shot?

So? You need five injections of DPT and a tetanus booster every 10 years.

Vaccines for Hepatitis B and Hepatitis A

The hepatitis B vaccine, or "hep B" as it is commonly referred to, has been routine in all 50 states now for several years. It is a series of three shots that is begun in the hospital before a newborn is discharged and is followed up by two more shots in the first year of life. The killed vaccine is specific for preventing liver infection by the type B hepatitis virus. Since the series is begun in the hospital as a part of routine newborn care, most parents of newborns do not object to completing the series, and I don't get a lot of questions about hepatitis B from them. It is the parents whose unvaccinated children are of school age who have the questions.

What is hepatitis B?

The hepatitis B virus causes serious liver disease resulting in jaundice (yellow skin) and extreme debilitation. It can last for months and in some cases can cause death. It also has the potential to remain in the liver forever and cause chronic mild to moderate illness; it can lead to cirrhosis (liver scarring), liver cancer, and death. It is very serious and there is no adequate treatment. We are fortunate to have a vaccine against hepatitis B virus.

How do you catch hepatitis B?

The hepatitis B virus is spread by blood and other infectious bodily fluids such as semen and even sweat. You can get it from sharing dirty needles or having sex with infected people. I know of at least one case where it was passed during a wrestling match. It is unlikely that it can be spread by sweat, saliva, urine, or stool unless there is blood on the skin or in the mouth, urinary tract, or gastrointestinal tract (you just never know). It is passed from a mother to her fetus. It is relatively easily passed from person to person as compared with the virus that causes AIDS. Intimate contact is not necessary.

My children are older and were not vaccinated at birth. Why do they have to be vaccinated? We don't know anyone with hepatitis B and they are too young to have sex or take drugs.

Their risk for hepatitis B is low now; however, as they approach adolescence, their risk greatly increases. Get them vaccinated now while you still have some control and can make sure they complete the whole series of three shots. How do you know that you don't know anyone with hepatitis B?

I think I would know if someone had a serious liver disease!

Really? We in the United States have been lucky that hepatitis B has been largely confined to high-risk groups such as hemophiliacs, homosexuals, prostitutes, and drug abusers. However, in many other countries of the world, especially in Asia, most people have been exposed to hepatitis B. They pass it around to each other through "traditional" sexual contact and to their children during pregnancy. Many Asians are exposed and infected from birth. They have more tolerance to it than we do (almost as if they are "vaccinated") and have less serious illness than we do. To them, it is a routine childhood illness. Some of their children may be playing with yours at recess or during physical education.

Okay, I'll get them vaccinated. Then I can forget all about hepatitis, right?

Wrong. You can forget all about hepatitis B, but there are still other forms of hepatitis you still have to worry about.

Why's that?

"Hepatitis" is just a general term that means inflammation of the liver. It can be caused by many viruses, drugs such as alcohol or Tylenol (in overdose), or other noninfectious disease states. Hepatitis B is just one of many (six or seven at last count) viruses that *primarily* affect the liver. We only have vaccines for hepatitis A and B, not hepatitis C, D, E, or the others. There are also many other viruses (such as the Epstein-Barr virus that causes mononucleosis or the varicella-zoster virus that causes chickenpox) whose primary target is not the liver but they have the potential to wreak havoc there. However, just because a vaccine doesn't cover everything under the sun is no reason not to get it. Be glad that there's one for hepatitis B because it is a bad actor.

What is hepatitis A?

Hepatitis A is another virus that affects the liver. It is spread hand to mouth and is epidemic where there are unsanitary conditions (e.g., day care and third-world countries). It is easily passed hand to mouth from one person to another via contact with stool (toilets, doorknobs, and diaper pails).

It is not serious and may be unrecognized in children or manifest itself as just another "stomach virus." However, it can make older children and adults very sick, even jaundiced, for a couple of weeks. Recovery is usually complete and there are no serious long-term sequelae. The vaccine is recommended for anyone who wants to avoid hepatitis A infection and high-risk populations.

Miscellaneous Immunization Questions

Is it safe to give immunizations when a child is ill?

Most of the time, yes. Vaccines can be given safely when a child has a typical mild viral illness. The immune response to the vaccine is unaffected. However, if the child's illness is still evolving and the diagnosis is uncertain, it may be best to postpone the immunizations so as not to confuse the picture of the underlying illness. Since chickenpox and influenza are known to cause some relative immunosuppression, most pediatricians will not administer vaccines to a child who might have chickenpox or influenza. Since there are many children who don't get regular medical care except when they are ill, this may be the only opportunity to vaccinate them.

My doctor always makes me bring my child back for a "well check" before giving the vaccinations. Why?

This is more likely a scheduling decision than a medical one. Preparing and administering vaccines take a lot of nursing time that may be needed for "sick" child care. More time is allotted for well checks to handle immunizations. If the doctor thinks the patient may not return for the immunizations, they are administered at a "sick" visit if they can be given safely.

What's the difference between Hib and hep B?

Haemophilus influenzae type B, or Hib, is a vaccine against a bacteria that used to be the number one cause of serious invasive infections in young children (e.g., meningitis). Hep B is the vaccine against one of the many viruses that can cause hepatitis, which can lead to chronic, debilitating disease, cancer, and death. It is passed in the same ways but much more easily than the AIDS virus.

Can the pertussis vaccine cause seizures and brain damage?

All current scientific evidence argues against pertussis (also known as whooping cough) vaccine being responsible for seizures and brain damage. Pertussis infection and its potential complications, however, can result in seizures and brain damage. Pertussis is still very much a concern.

What is this new DTaP?

It is a newer version of the DPT vaccine that has an improved version of the pertussis component. It confers protection with less side effects such as fever and fussiness.

Why do we now need a second dose of MMR vaccine?

A lesson was learned here. As more people became immune to measles through immunization and not natural infection, there were very few cases of natural measles around, although it was not eradicated. The immunity provided by immunization was not as long lasting as the immunity from natural infection, and immunity was not naturally boosted through occasional contact with wild (natural) measles virus.

Although this was not unexpected, there were no epidemics and things seemed to be working well even with the shorter lived immunity provided by immunization. However, the "herd" still had a lot of people in it who were immune because of natural infection.

Nowadays the "herd" is comprised mostly of individuals who are immune due to vaccination. The critical number of susceptible individuals was exceeded and we saw our first epidemics. Now a second shot is needed.

Couldn't the same thing happen with chickenpox vaccine?

This may turn out to be the case with chickenpox vaccine. Studies are under way, but there's no need to delay the first immunization just in case a second one may be needed later on.

Do you really need a tetanus shot every 10 years?

Yes, but there's time to get one if you have an injury and have reasonable access to medical care.

What is the Pneumovax?

Pneumococci are bacteria (dozens actually) that are responsible for many serious and not so serious invasive infections—ear infections, sinusitis, pneumonia, and meningitis to name a few. The vaccine is effective for about 20 of the many varieties and does not work for children under the age of 2 years. It may be a good idea for a child who suffers frequent ear and sinus infections or has other underlying medical conditions. Scientists are working on a vaccine that covers more of the strains and that can be given to even younger children.

What changes in immunization can we look forward to?

A simplified immunization schedule using more combination vaccines, vaccines that can be given intranasally or with foods, vaccines for diarrhea-causing *Rotavirus* and pneumonia-causing respiratory syncytial virus (RSV), vaccines for herpesviruses and neonatal *Streptococcus,* and a vaccine for AIDS.

Glossary

acetaminophen   A medication to reduce pain and fever. It does not affect inflammation.

acquired immune deficiency syndrome (AIDS)   No longer really a syndrome now that the cause is known to be the human immunodeficiency virus. A fatal illness (at this writing) caused by a virus that destroys critical parts of the immune system, resulting in an inability to prevent infection and destroy cancer cells. It is passed via blood and sexual contact.

acyclovir   An antiviral drug that specifically "cripples" but does not kill herpesviruses. Also known as Zovirax.

albuterol   The generic name of a drug that dilates (enlarges) the airways of the lungs; also commonly known as Ventolin or Proventil. Comes in a liquid or a pill or in a cannister or a sterile vial for inhalation. This drug is the mainstay of treatment for asthma. The most common side effects are jitteriness and rapid heartbeat. Asthmatics should not leave home without it.

alveoli   Plural of alveolus, a tiny air sac at the end of the smallest airway in the lungs where the actual exchange of oxygen and carbon dioxide occurs. These sacs fill with fluid during bacterial pneumonias.

amino acids   The "building blocks" of proteins, which along with fats and carbohydrates, vitamins, and minerals account for all the types of molecules found in the body.

amphetamine   A central and peripheral nervous system stimulant drug.

antibiotic   A drug used to fight bacterial infection.

antihistamine   Allergy medication to counteract the effect of histamine.

aphthous stomatitis   Recurrent, painful mouth ulcers on the gums, cheeks, and tongue; its cause is unknown, but there is a strong hereditary factor.

bacteria   Single-celled infectious agents.

bell curve   A statistical graph that is shaped like a bell. Average occurs along the height of the bell and the extremes on the shorter ends of the bell. It's a way of showing that the average occurs most frequently and the extremes rarely.

bilirubin   A pigment formed from the breakdown of hemoglobin that can tinge the skin yellow.

blood incompatibility   When two different blood types are mixed and try to destroy each other.

BRAT diet   A diet of bananas, rice, applesauce, and toast. A time-honored diet for those who have gastrointestinal illness. There's nothing magic about it and it should not be followed religiously for more than a day or two. Add new foods as fast as tolerated. The diet is not recommended for anyone who doesn't like bananas, rice, applesauce, or toast or anyone who would prefer to eat just about anything else.

bronchi   Plural of bronchus, which is a large major airway that branches off the trachea and leads to the lung. Smaller divisions of the airways are known as bronchioles. Bronchodilation and bronchoconstriction refer to enlargement and shrinking, respectively, of the diameter of the bronchi and bronchioles.

Candida   The most common kind of yeast that can cause thrush and diaper rash in infants.

cathartic   A substance that moves and empties the bowels.

catheter   A small plastic tube that can be inserted into any orifice. In office pediatrics it is most commonly used to collect urine.

cholesterol   A steroid molecule made in the liver and absorbed from the diet that is important in the synthesis of steroid hormones such as cortisol, testosterone, progesterone, and estrogen and is a major component of bile.

chromosome   DNA-containing structures found in the nucleus of a cell that are responsible for reproducing genetic information.

congenital   Present at birth, which probably means present during fetal life as well.

congestion   Dilation of blood vessels.

conjunctivitis   Inflammation of the transparent membrane that covers the white part of the eye.

dander   Allergen dispersed into the environment by furry and feathery animals consisting of dead skin cells, hair, feathers, and saliva.

debride   Remove foreign material and contaminated and dead tissue.

decongestant   A medication that shrinks blood vessels.

dermatitis   Inflammation of the skin.

diphtheria   A bacterial infection that results in a swollen throat and subsequent airway obstruction.

DNA   Deoxyribonucleic acid; the double-helix molecule that is the blueprint for all genetic information.

DPT or DTP   A combination vaccine for diphtheria, pertussis, and tetanus. It has no live components.

eczema   Another word for dermatitis or inflammation of the skin.

electrocardiogram (ECG)   An electrical tracing of the heart; also called EKG.

emetic   A substance that induces vomiting.

Emetrol   Brand name of an over-the-counter preparation that is meant to suppress vomiting.

ENT   Ears, nose, throat; a physician who specializes in the treatment of the ears, nose, and throat. Some subspecialize in *pediatric* ENT diseases. Most adult ENTs will see children, but pediatric ENTs do not usually see adults.

epinephrine   Commonly known as adrenaline, it is the "fight or flight" hormone that revs up the body in the face of threatening situations. It increases the heart rate and blood pressure, opens up the airways, diverts blood from the gastrointestinal tract to the muscles, and raises the blood sugar. It is released quickly and dissipates quickly, causing a "rush" followed by a period of feeling "spent."

EpiPen, EpiPen Jr.   A single, preprepared dose of epinephrine (adrenaline) for immediate injection into the muscle of persons with a serious or potentially serious allergic reaction. Anyone who has a history of allergic reactions should carry this drug or have it immediately available. It can be lifesaving. It is *not* to be used in lieu of, but *in addition* to, a trip to the emergency department.

Epstein-Barr (EB) virus   Responsible for infectious mononucleosis; a member of the herpesvirus family.

esophagus   The tube in the throat in which food travels to the stomach. It lies behind the windpipe (trachea).

expectorant   An agent that promotes the ejection of mucus from the lungs or trachea by decreasing its viscosity.

febrile seizure "Febrile" is the adjective form of "fever," as in febrile illness or febrile seizure. The seizure (convulsion) is usually associated
with fever.

formulary A list of approved medications and other medical supplies.
Since many medications are very similar, hospitals and other institutions limit a physician's choice to keep costs down.

full term Refers to a pregnancy that lasts 37 to 40 weeks. The closer to 40
weeks, the "fuller" the term, but pregnancies lasting at least 37 weeks
qualify as term.

fungus Type of primitive plant capable of causing infection, usually in
patients with relative immunosuppression.

gene Section of a chromosome whose action contributes to a specific inherited trait.

genitourinary The sexual and urinary organs.

gingivostomatitis Inflammation of the gums and mouth; in pediatrics
this term refers to herpesvirus infection in young children characterized by very high fever, red, swollen gums, and mouth ulcers.

gland A term that broadly includes any aggregation of specialized cells
that secrete or excrete a product; usually refers to the strategically
placed lymph nodes that enlarge in the presence of infection.

griseofulvin A drug used to treat fungal infections. Its use must be monitored carefully since it typically is given for a period of several weeks
and has the potential to cause serious side effects such as liver damage
and low blood counts.

guaifenesin An over-the-counter medication that is supposed to improve
the flow of mucous secretions in the lungs so that they can be coughed
up. It is often found in cough and cold medications in combination
with a cough suppressant

hemoglobin The molecule in red blood cells that is responsible for carry-
ing oxygen. A large part of it is iron.

hemophiliacs Persons, usually male, with the tendency to bleed uncontrollably. This disease can be adequately treated with infusion of special blood clotting factors derived from the blood of healthy donors.

hep B Abbreviation for the vaccine against hepatitis type B, a virus that
infects the liver.

hepatitis Inflammation of the liver from any cause.

herpesviruses A large class of viruses. Infection by herpesviruses is
asymptomatic in most cases, but they are also responsible for illnesses

such as chickenpox, shingles, gingivostomatitis, cold sores, genital sores, mononucleosis, and roseola. May be responsible for many of the "viral syndromes" characterized by fever, fussiness, rash, and seizures in infants.

Hib　Abbreviation for the vaccine against *Haemophilus influenzae* type b, a bacterium that caused significant invasive illness in children (e.g., meningitis and pneumonia) before a vaccine was developed.

high-risk individuals　Persons who are, have been, or potentially can become immunocompromised and thus are more prone to serious illness, persons who choose to place themselves in unusual jeopardy rendering them more susceptible to serious illness (health care workers, snake tamers, sword swallowers, etc.), persons who are in unusually close quarters and in contact with many people (institutions, day care centers, boarding schools, nursing homes, hospitals, space shuttles). It's a very long list and most everyone can be considered high risk to some degree so it can be a judgment call.

hives　Allergic response of the skin characterized by redness, itching, swelling, and often the presence of welts that can come and go quickly.

hormone　A substance released by a gland into the blood that has actions elsewhere in the body.

hydrocortisone cream, 1%　A very mild steroid cream available over the counter that has anti-inflammatory properties. It is mostly used for itching and red, dry skin or bug bites. Cortaid and many other generic brands are available. A half-strength preparation of hydrocortisone cream (0.5%) is also available.

hypersensitivity　A more accurate term for what is commonly referred to as allergy. Allergy implies that some physical irritant provokes the response; hypersensitivity implies that the response is unwarranted. In many allergic conditions no physical irritant can be identified, but the body reacts as if one is present (i.e., it is hypersensitive).

ibuprofen　A type of nonsteroidal anti-inflammatory medication.

immune surveillance　"Patrolling" by the immune system, being vigilant for breaks in security.

immune system　A complex system that protects the body by resisting infection, disease, toxic substances, and any other real or imagined threat. In its broadest sense it can include the skin (a protective barrier) and brain *(run away!)*. More specifically, it includes protective reflexes such as itching, coughing, and vomiting. Most specifically, it includes specialized cells that manufacture and release chemicals that promote resistance and healing.

immunologically mediated Caused and controlled by the immune system. Refers to a process that is the direct result of the body trying to protect itself rather than the result of a specific intruder. Many more previously misunderstood illnesses are now being determined to be immunologically mediated, that is, the result of a security force run amok; we've gotten "too good" at defending ourselves.

immunosuppression, immunocompromised, relative immunosuppression These terms refer to less than optimal functioning of any or all parts of the immune system. Some causes are fatigue and stress, drugs such as steroids or alcohol, congenital defects (remember the "bubble boy"?), prematurity or Down syndrome, preceding illness such as influenza, tuberculosis, cancer, radiation therapy, drug abuse, AIDS, old age, newborn status, pregnancy, heart disease, lung disease, kidney disease, liver disease, gastrointestinal disease, diabetes and other glandular diseases, blood diseases, bone diseases, and brain diseases. *Anything* that results in a decreased ability to defend the body can result in a state of relative immunosuppression. Depending on the cause, the degree and duration of immunosuppression can vary from mild and temporary to life threatening and lifelong.

Imodium A-D An over-the counter medication that is used to treat diarrhea by paralyzing the gut. It is not recommended in the early stages of a diarrheal illness.

inflammation Process through which the body heals itself; it is signaled by warmth, swelling, redness, drainage, pain, and tenderness.

IV fluids Intravenous (into the vein) administration of a solution of water, sugar, and salt.

jaundice Yellow discoloration of the skin due to the pigment bilirubin, a product of hemoglobin breakdown.

ketoconazole A drug used to treat fungal infections. Its use must be monitored carefully since it it is generally given for a period of several weeks and has the potential to cause serious side effects such as liver damage, particularly when used with other drugs processed in the liver (e.g., erythromycin and alcohol).

lactose/lactase A sugar (lactose) that is composed of two simpler sugars, glucose and galactose. It is broken down into glucose and galactose by an enzyme (lactase) in the intestine.

larynx   The voicebox; it is found within the trachea. When it is swollen, it is called laryngitis and the voice is hoarse and the cough is croupy.

measles   A highly infectious viral illness characterized by a red rash, fever, and severe cough; also known as rubeola.

meningitis   The most feared pediatric infectious illness. It refers to inflammation of the lining that covers the brain and spinal cord (the meninges). The most common causes of this inflammation are bacteria and viruses, although there are other rare causes. It can lead to brain damage to varying degrees. Diagnosis is made by a spinal tap (sticking a needle into the back and withdrawing fluid).

MMR   Measles, mumps, rubella; a live, attenuated vaccine.

morbidity   Disability caused by disease.

mucosa   Specialized moist "skin" that lines the mouth, nose, throat, ears, vagina, eyes, etc.; also called mucous membrane.

mucous membranes   The mucosa, the wet lining of orifices such as the mouth, nose, eyes, and genitals.

mumps   A viral illness primarily affecting the salivary glands of the cheeks.

narcotic   A drug that induces a stuporous state (insensibility) and relieves pain. Commonly refers to drugs such as morphine, heroin, and codeine that are both physically and psychologically addictive. Narcotics have a tendency to suppress breathing in young children and in cases of overdose.

natural selection   A term coined by Charles Darwin to describe the principle whereby environmental factors act to inhibit the survival of some species, thereby indirectly promoting the survival of other species. This mechanism aids in the "survival of the fittest."

NIX   An over-the-counter creme hair conditioner that contains a drug that kills head lice and its eggs (nits).

nonsteroidal anti-inflammatory drugs (NSAIDs)   Medications that suppress inflammation that do not have the structure of a steroid molecule nor the usual side effects of steroids. Most commonly used to describe drugs such as ibuprofen (Motrin) but includes aspirin and cromolyn and others.

nuclear scan   An imaging technique that uses radioactively labeled molecules injected into a vein to produce a picture.

nystatin   An anti-yeast medication commonly used to treat thrush and diaper rashes in babies caused by yeast *(Candida)*.

over the counter (OTC)   Refers to medications that can be bought at drug and grocery stores without a prescription.

pain   An unpleasant sensation of discomfort of varying degrees.

pathology   Disease.

Pedialyte   Brand name for a fluid commonly used to maintain hydration in sick infants. It is composed of sugar, salt, and water.

pertussis   A bacterial infection known as whooping cough; it is the "P" and "aP" in the DTP and DTaP vaccine. Pertussis is a bad, lingering cold with cough in older children and adults, but it can be life threatening in young infants. The most vulnerable infants are usually those *younger than 2 months* of age who cannot be vaccinated successfully. This is a good example of "herd immunity" protecting these newborn infants.

phototherapy   A treatment involving exposing the skin of jaundiced babies to light rays to decrease their bilirubin levels.

placebo   Any treatment that offers relief even if there is no scientific evidence that it should do so. The "placebo effect" is very powerful, which proves how important the brain is in the immune system.

pneumococcal   Pertaining to the bacterium *Streptococcus pneumoniae* of which there are dozens of subtypes.

polio   A viral illness that produces fever, headache, sore throat, and vomiting. In some cases it can involve the nervous system and cause stiff neck and back; in the most severe cases it causes permanent deformity and paralysis.

prophylactic   Protective.

pus   A liquid inflammatory product consisting mostly of infection-fighting white blood cells.

rectum   The terminal part of the intestinal tract that ends at the anal opening.

respiratory depression   Decrease in the inherent drive to breathe resulting in fewer breaths per minute.

respiratory distress   Inability to breathe adequately resulting in a feeling of air hunger and usually more breaths per minute.

respiratory syncytial virus (RSV)   Common respiratory virus that includes many strains. Causes cold symptoms in most people but can cause more severe and potentially life-threatening wheezing and respiratory distress in very small or young infants or in immunocompromised children. There is no cure and treatment is supportive. Vaccines offer promise in the future.

Reye's syndrome Frequently fatal illness that involves the liver and brain. Its cause is unknown, but it has been associated with the use of aspirin during episodes of influenza or chickenpox. Since aspirin is rarely used during childhood illnesses anymore, Reye's syndrome is now a rarity.

rhinitis Inflammation of the mucosal lining of the nose, usually due to colds or allergy.

roseola A viral illness caused by a herpesvirus that usually occurs around the age of 6 to 12 months. It is characterized by 3 to 5 days of high temperature and occasionally a runny nose and fussiness, followed by resolution of the fever and the appearance of a diffuse pink rash.

Rotavirus Also known as "winter vomiting virus," a common virus that is responsible for many of the more severe cases of gastrointestinal illness. Frequently is epidemic in families, day care centers, and communities. Can cause high temperature lasting up to 5 days, persistent vomiting, and prolonged diarrhea, which result in dehydration in small children. Vaccines are being developed.

rubella A mild viral illness resulting in a pink rash in most cases, but when contracted in the first trimester of pregnancy, it can cause serious birth defects; also known as German measles.

screening urinalysis A routine test of a urine sample when there is no evidence to suggest that there is any kind of a urinary problem.

self-limiting Resolves on its own, usually after a predictable course.

shingles A painful skin condition caused by the re-emergence of the virus that caused an earlier case of chickenpox.

sign Objective evidence of disease that is recognized or elicited by the physician.

sonogram A noninvasive imaging study that uses sound waves to produce a picture.

standard of care What physicians are *expected* to do in a particular situation; usually but not always the *best* thing to do.

streptococcal (strep) Refers to the bacterium *Streptococcus* that can cause infection anywhere but is most commonly used to describe throat infection. There are hundreds of types and strains.

sudden infant death syndrome (SIDS) An enigma characterized by infants unexpectedly dying in their sleep from no known cause. Most commonly occurs between 6 weeks and 9 months of age. It probably has many causes, but the most significant may be a genetic predisposition to stop breathing that is aggravated by being placed face down to sleep. Since babies are now put to sleep on their backs, the incidence of

SIDS has decreased. Other risk factors may include maternal smoking, low birth weight, lower socioeconomic class, and upper respiratory symptoms.

supportive treatment   Treatment of individual symptoms as they occur when there is no cure for the underlying illness.

suppository   A solid medication that is meant to be dissolved in the rectum.

surveillance testing   Careful sampling of the community to monitor types and activities of disease-causing agents.

symptom   Subjective evidence of disease that is recognized by the patient.

syndrome   A set of symptoms that commonly occur together without a known underlying cause. Once the cause is known, the illness is usually renamed in such a way as to identify its cause; for example, most professionals no longer say AIDS but HIV for human immunodeficiency virus.

tenderness   An unpleasant sensation of discomfort of varying degrees elicited only when pressure is applied to the affected site.

tetanus   An infection by a bacterium found in dirt whose neurotoxin can produce "lockjaw" and subsequent airway obstruction.

thrush   Yeast infection of the oral mucosa.

topical   Applied to the surface of, for example onto the skin, into the eyes, or into the nose.

trachea   The windpipe; it traverses the neck and chest and lies in front of the esophagus (the tube that food goes down).

tuberculosis   A bacterial infection primarily of the lung that can then spread to any organ of the body.

urethra   The urinary tract between the bladder and the outside of the body.

varicella   Chickenpox.

varicella-zoster virus   The virus responsible for chickenpox and shingles; a member of the herpesvirus family.

Varivax   Vaccine for the varicella-zoster virus that causes chickenpox.

Vermox   A drug that kills many human parasites; in pediatrics it is most often used to treat pinworms. One pill is given to each family member and a second pill is given 2 weeks later. There are no significant side effects.

viral syndrome A set of symptoms that commonly occur together under similar circumstances that are presumed to be due to an unnamed virus because of the nature of the symptoms. Symptoms commonly last several days and can include fever, fussiness, irritability, decreased appetite, diarrhea, vomiting, and rash.

virus Minute infectious agent that can reproduce only in living host cells.

wheezing A subtle whistling sound heard with a stethoscope in patients who have airflow obstruction in the lower airways of the lungs.

yeast A type of fungus that thrives in dark, warm, wet places. They reside on the mucous membranes of everyone but only grow uncontrollably and cause problems during periods of relative immunosuppression.

zoster Shingles.

Index